KUM NYE
TIBETAN YOGA

KUM NYE

— TIBETAN YOGA —

TARTHANG TULKU

DHARMA PUBLISHING INTERNATIONAL

Other Kum Nye Yoga titles by Tarthang Tulku:
Tibetan Relaxation; Kum Nye massage and movement
Full color ill., 135 pp., ISBN 0-89800-346-6
*The Joy of Being; Kum Nye practices for relaxation, integration
and concentration* 310 pp., ISBN 0-89800-388-1

Editing and illustration by Dharma Publishing
Typeset in DTL Albertina and Linotype Syntax,
printed and bound by Dharma Press, California
Cover design and layout by Colin Dorsey

Library of Congress Control Number 2006939217
ISBN ISBN-13: 978 089800-421-2   2
      ISBN-10: 0-89800-421-7

9 8 7 6 5 4 3 2 1

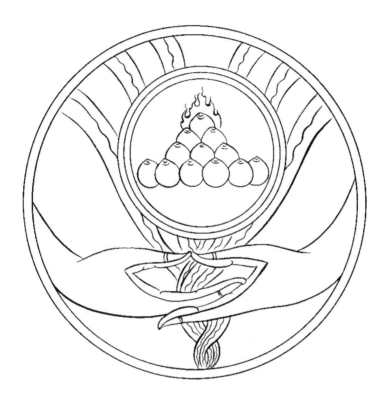

Body, mind and senses join
through a process of inner alchemy

Table of Contents

Foreword to this edition

It is with pleasure that I received the request of Arnaud Maitland of Dharma Publishing to offer a few words on the occasion of this reprint of Kum Nye Relaxation. For the convenience of readers, this new edition offers the two original volumes combined in a single publication.

Since first introducing Kum Nye in America over thirty-five years ago, I have seen it bring benefits to many individuals. Mind and body both seem to need relaxation, especially in today's world where the busyness of everyday activities generates much stress. With Kum Nye, we can loosen up the tension connected with this stress and open up the sensitivity inherent in our human embodiment.

By tuning and refining this sensitivity each day, we can make progress in releasing our being from constrictions that prevent us from actively engaging ourselves. This releasing and refinement immediately bring an enriching quality into our lives, while gradually leading us toward the spiritual path. Regularly engaging in Kum Nye prepares the ground for meditation and helps create the conditions that allow one to become a candidate for serious Dharma study and practice.

I would like to take this opportunity to thank Dharma Publishing and all the international teachers of Kum Nye around the world for making access to these teachings available to a wide audience.

Tarthang Tulku
Odiyan, October 2006

Preface

Relaxation is a gentle healing system that relieves stress, transforms negative patterns, helps us to be more balanced and healthy, and increases our enjoyment and apreciation of life. In these times when confusion and chaos are a part of daily activity, we are often too tense and charged up to enjoy life. Kum Nye opens our senses and our hearts so that we feel satisfied and fulfilled and can appreciate more fully every aspect of our lives. Even in a short time, the quality of experience can be enriched and our lives grow more harmonious.

The unique value of the Kum Nye system of relaxation is that it integrates and balances two approaches, the physical and the psychological. Kum Nye heals both our bodies and minds, bringing their energies together to function calmly and smoothly. As it leads to the integration of body and mind in all our activities, this relaxation has a vital and lasting quality greater than the feeling of well-being experienced in physical exercise, or even in disciplines such as yoga. When we learn to open our senses and touch our feelings directly, our bodies and minds make contact with one another, and all experience becomes rich, healthy, and more beautiful. As we become deeply

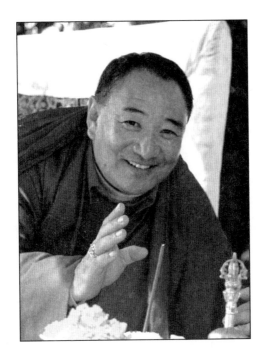

acquainted with ourselves and our self-understanding grows, we are also able to share more fully with others.

The written tradition of Kum Nye is contained in medical Tibetan texts, as well as in the ancient Vinaya texts of Buddhism. These texts deal with living to physical and universal laws, and include extensive descriptions of healing practices. Kum Nye (pronounced *Koom Nyay*) is thus part of the lineage of spiritual and medical theories and practices which links Tibetan with Indian and Chinese medicine. This lineage has given rise to many disciplines, including yoga and acupuncture; it also forms the roots of many of the more recent body-mind disciplines.

Yet the system of Kum Nye presented in this book is
thoroughly modern, drawn from my own experience, and
adapted specifically to suit modern needs. When I was a
young boy in Tibet, my father, who was a physician and a
lama, introduced me to Kum Nye. Kum Nye, however, not
well known in Tibet, was most often used as an adjunct
to other practices. My gurus in the oral introductory yoga
tradition of the Nying-thig tsa-lung (subtle body energy system) sometimes taught the basic theory and practice of
Kum Nye as an introductory practice. Kum Nye has had
no systematized body of written instructions until now,
and my practice of Kum Nye had a flavor of exploration
and experimentation.

I have used this open aspect of Kum Nye to make further adaptations. Over the past decades, I have developed
several hundred exercises which my Western students
have found particularly helpful. These volumes include
the simplest and most effective of these exercises, all of
which can be done safely—by young and old—without
a teacher. Breathing, self-massage, and different kinds of
movement exercises are included. I hope that delight in the
discovery of many as yet undeveloped aspects of Kum Nye
will enrich the practice of Western students, and eventually encourage systematization in Western terms.

I hope this book will introduce the benefits of Kum
Nye to many people of various backgrounds and interests,

and will assist them in developing and continuing their experience of inner relaxation. I intended the book to be a practical guide to the pleasure of a healthy and balanced life, rich in beauty and enjoyment, and leading to harmony for all beings, even in these difficult times.

I am grateful to the many whose experience of Kum Nye has contributed to the development of these exercises. I dedicate this book to the Nyingma Institute in Berkeley, California, where Kum Nye grew and blossomed in its present form.

Tarthang Tulku,
September 1978

Exercises and Massages

XIV

PART TWO: MOVEMENT EXERCISES

Balancing and Integrating: Stage One

Balancing and Integrating: Stage Two

EXERCISES AND MASSAGES

Part One

THEORY, PREPARATION, MASSAGE

The Inner and Outer Massage of Feeling

Through relaxation we discover a whole new way of being.

We all have memories of times when we felt particularly alive, when the world seemed fresh and promising, like a flower garden on a bright spring morning. Whatever the circumstances leading to such moments, there is suddenly a sensation of acute vitality supported by the knowledge that all elements are in absolute harmony. The air pulses with life. Our bodies feel healthy and energetic, our minds clear and confident. There is a lucent quality to perception. Every feature of the environment pleases the senses: colors are vivid, sounds melodious, and odors fragrant. All aspects of the experience blend perfectly and there is a vibrant quality to everything; the usual border between inner and outer space becomes fluid. Nothing is fixed, and we feel spacious and open. We act with perfect ease and appropriateness.

The essence of this experience is balance, and its offshoot is a deep feeling of nurturance and refreshment which extends far beyond the feeling we would call 'happiness'. Kum Nye is the art of developing this true balance. Through relaxation we can discover a new way of being, a perspective that is open and that delights in the integration of body, mind, senses, feelings, and environment. We learn to appreciate the completely wholesome quality of *living* experience. The whole body becomes refreshed, as if showered within by pure spring water. Not only the physical body quickens, but the mind and all of the senses are invigorated as well; sense impressions and thoughts come to life. A quality of relaxation informs every activity, even walking or eating. Our lives function smoothly, and we become healthy and balanced.

The key to both our internal integration and a balanced relationship with the world lies within our feelings and sensations. We can nurture and heal both our bodies and minds by touching our feelings deeply and expanding the flowing rhythms they bring to us, for they are linked to the vitality of the universe itself. Through relaxation, we awaken feelings which then expand and accumulate until we slowly become aware of a deep, interpenetrating field of energy, inside our body and beyond it. This energy can stimulate itself internally to sustain and nurture us in our daily lives, recycling sensation so we become sensitive and strong, and our sensations rich and powerful. Our minds become clearer as well, and we discover what it means to be balanced.

Our senses, feelings, and thoughts are integrated, and all of our relationships, actions, ideas, and movements are flowing and harmonious. Our awareness gives us the freedom to take charge of our lives, not in a forceful or grasping way, but with confidence. We then naturally do what is appropriate and beneficial, and function in a positive way in the world. We realize that ideas and actions which result in stability and happiness for ourselves contribute also to the harmony of the world around us.

When we sense the beauty of the world, it seems natural to live in harmony with the universe, to enjoy a mutually satisfying relationship like a mare and her foal. But somehow we have become estranged from this state of being. Though we speak of Mother Nature, we are like her adolescent children, struggling with our own identities at the cost of losing the warmth and gentleness we vaguely remember.

In early childhood, when our senses were more open, we may have experienced a greater sense of union with the universe, but as we grow, we learn to foster our personalities too intensely, deepening feelings of separation rather than the feelings of warmth and security our hearts desire. The pressures and complications of modern society make it difficult to do otherwise, for to be successful in business, in friendship, even in play, we are almost forced into competitive and stressful situations which develop feelings of alienation and anxiety. All our major undertakings, including school, raising a family, and becoming established in a career, involve complications and limitations we cannot seem to avoid.

Even when we try to open our lives, we may end up contracting our experience rather than expanding it. Our mental and physical activities seldom succeed in truly satisfying us, because we do not integrate the two. Not realizing the importance of integrating body and mind in *all* our activities, we emphasize mental achievement at the expense of feeling, or our physical body at the expense of the rich sensations within.

When we restrict our feelings and sensations, we prevent them from giving us the sustenance we need to be healthy and happy. Our senses may react to this constriction and subtly urge us to open, but our 'rational' mind is in control of delicate sense impressions, and so we may not even hear their plea. Hungry for fulfillment, we begin to search outside ourselves, often racing restlessly from one source of enjoyment to another, as if there were a limited supply. We are captivated by the idea that satisfaction is 'out there' . . . only we look, work, or play hard enough. We are drawn to exciting activities which seem to stimulate our minds and senses, but leave us still wanting more. The faster we run, the further we move away from true satisfaction, which remains within, behind the door of the senses.

Instead of opening this door, we may turn to drugs such as alcohol or the hallucinogens. We may even turn to the spiritual path, hoping at last to be truly nurtured, only to discover that here, too, we are still dissatisfied.

We continue to expend our energies jumping from experience to experience, from thought to thought. We imagine what we would like to have happen, or remember what it was like before; we make plans. Lost in daydreams, we may glimpse a moment of pleasure or a rich sensation, but we do not experience the full flavor of the contact; somehow it eludes us.

We may attempt to regain a feeling of wholeness by 'ownership' of our families and of property, trying in this way to control both nature and our lives. But such control is artificial and out of touch with the natural laws and cycles which govern our bodies and minds, as well as the world around us. We begin to feel closed in and unfulfilled. Unable to see that our lack of balance might have been the cause, we find ourselves in unhealthy situations, wondering how we got there.

We may believe that it is impossible for us to perceive things more substantially or to open into deeper levels of experience. Through neglect, our senses have toughened like an elephant's hide, diminishing the fullness of our sensory capacity. Until we gently soften this 'toughness' by developing the natural energies of our feelings and sensations, we cannot open to the full field of experience.

When we really *know* this, we can participate in the natural flow of the universe, for we understand that we depend on nature, and nature, indeed the whole universe, depends on us. The world will be balanced when we are balanced. We are naturally bonded to the world: the elements which make up the universe are within each of us. We carry this ancient lineage in our bodies, and we are reflected in our families, our society, and our planet. Every action we take, however small, affects the whole universe, just as every wave affects the shore.

We participate in infinitely complex and interdependent relationships with all of the many levels of existence, from subatomic to cosmic. Like other systems in the universe, we are a complete unit in ourselves, yet we are composed of many smaller units which are all interrelated and which also interrelate with the whole. In addition to the many systems that make up the physical body—skeletal, muscular, nervous, etcetera—there is the psychological or emotional system as well as other subtle energy systems. The functioning of these systems depends on the functioning of every other system in the body, while the state of the entire unit we call the 'human being' is intimately related to the condition of the environment.

Our immediate environment is also related to every other environment on earth, and the earth is influenced by events in the far reaches of the universe. We are influenced by many forces, some of which we barely perceive or understand. Our actions and thoughts affect other systems, including microscopic worlds within our bodies.

When we acknowledge these interrelationships, we acknowledge the importance of creating harmony within ourselves. We realize that we have the resources we need to be both balanced and happy, for our bodies and minds are the vehicles for all our learning and growth. By slowing down, relaxing, and opening the senses, we can learn to develop these resources. We then discover that we can heal our bodies and minds with feeling channeled through the physical body. When we lessen the chronic tightness in our muscles and minds, we sensitize ourselves to subtle qualities of feeling and bring them alive to vigorous and fresh experience, enriching them so they continue to grow like strong shoots.

As our mental and physical energies are vitalized and become integrated, these sensations become much more fertile and nurturing than ordinary sensations. Their nourishment frees us from the vibrant distraction of jumping thoughts and the wishing for what is always beyond our reach. We discover the virtually alert and flowing state of the body, mind, and energy, so we are able to find satisfaction within ourselves. As our bodies and minds become good friends, our muscles also work well together, free from superfluous muscle tension. We have the concentration necessary for full experience. Our relationships then become rich and deep, harmonious rather than competitive, for we relate more sensitively to others as well as to ourselves.

In Kum Nye there are various ways, including both stillness and movement, to stimulate the flow of feeling and energy that integrates body and mind. We begin by developing stillness of body, breath, and mind. Simply sitting still and relaxing gives us a chance to appreciate feelings of which we are normally unaware. Relaxation is then subtly aided by breathing through both nose and mouth, so gently and evenly that we are hardly conscious of inhaling and exhaling at all; a way of breathing which allows us to contact the positive vitality of the throat center.

As the breath becomes calm and quiet, fewer distracting thoughts and images run through the mind, and the whole body comes alive. Our mental and bodily energies become refreshed and tranquil, like a clear forest pool. We discover a quality of feeling common to body, breath, and mind—a calm, clear, deepening quality—soothing and 'massaging' us deep within. As we relax more, the subtle level of this feeling opens like a lens, letting in more 'light' or energy and creating comprehensive and more illuminating 'pictures' of experience.

To explore the qualities of this relaxation further, we add self-massage and the 'massage' of movement exercise to sitting and breathing. Usually we think of massage as something done for us, but the body can massage itself. Massage can involve our feelings and sensations and our whole inner structure, as well as our outer shape and form. During massage, subtle feeling-tones or energies permeate and soothe our whole being, integrating the mental and the physical, relating feeling to form. These energies are like a vibrating, moving aura which runs through us and outward from us, and also surrounds us. We can learn to heal ourselves inwardly with these energies, and direct them to flow outwardly, harmonizing all aspects of our being. We can generate an inner sun, radiating feelings that warm us and pervade everything around us.

While at first we stimulate the massage physically—by breathing, pressing and rubbing our bodies, moving very slowly in certain ways, or producing and releasing tension—later we can initiate massage through feeling-tones alone. As relaxation deepens, we begin to feel directly the interconnections among breath, senses, body, and mind. The senses open new channels and dimensions of sensation, releasing joyful feelings that expand and accumulate until we are aware of nothing else in the world. Every cell becomes suffused and saturated with positive feelings of wholeness and completion. Even between the muscles and tissues we drink in these wonderful feelings.

When we truly use our senses, every part of the body becomes alive and healthy—mentally and emotionally we become fully awake. We discover we can experience ecstatic beauty at every moment, as if we were always hearing beautiful music or seeing the finest works of art. We are even capable of healing ourselves, for this relaxation quickens a feeling-tone that itself becomes a self-generating massage, a system of self-nurturance that expands and develops. This is the massage of Kum Nye.

The deeper and richer our experience of this self-operating massage is, the more we will find that it simply can occur naturally, vitalizing every sense, feeling, and activity of daily life. Expanding in space and time, subtle feeling-tones or energies activate massage outside as well as inside our bodies, harmonizing surrounding levels of existence. Feelings of love or the joy of laughter expand beyond the body, floating through space and time like softly falling snow. The senses expand in a subtle way, increasing enjoyment.

When seeing, we lightly concentrate on an object so that we sense a feeling from its form. By opening our eyes in this way, we invite an ecstatic interaction between subtle 'inner' and 'outer' energies. Seeing then becomes vision, a constant expression of a vital totality.

Food becomes an offering to the senses. When we learn to enjoy all the feeling-tones of tasting, distributing them throughout the body and beyond it, eating is truly a meeting of the senses with their object, a ceremonial act of appreciation.

We learn to contact and appreciate sound as well, feeling it fully in our bodies, using it to stimulate harmonious interactions between ourselves and the surrounding universe. As we allow soft music to relax and soothe us when we are tired, we activate feelings which can even heal us. When we speak, each sound is gentle, so there is no shocking or destructive quality to our communication.

The sweetness bred by fully exercising our senses can be expanded more and more each day. Without trying to possess it, without any fixed goal, almost not caring, we let the joyful sensation come, opening our bodies to its gentle influence. Its quality, mild and sweet like milk and honey, touches us deeply, always continuing, refreshing itself, increasing until we enjoy an almost overwhelming feeling of fulfillment.

By breathing more subtly, we feel even more; a quality of softness intermixes with the warmth. Our bodies become light and still. Within the body and beyond it, subtle energies nourish feelings of satisfaction and harmony. We become integrated with these feelings, we are inseparable from them. Our awareness expands, relating many thoughts and feelings simultaneously and extending their duration. We discover the joy of exercising without effort. We live within a sense of freedom, a vital totality, a feeling which constantly accumulates. Life becomes a joyful flow in the universe: every cell, every sense, every part of consciousness past or future participates in this flow. In this way, we learn to live cheerfully. We will even live longer, for our lives are healthy and balanced.

As soon as the body and the breath are sufficiently calm and relaxed, immediately, almost magically, the joyful feeling arises. This is the feeling to expand and accumulate; this is the cream of Kum Nye, the essence. We can stir it so that it becomes richer and deeper, thick and vast. It can become so great it is almost everlasting, and we need never lose it. Its texture is creamy; its very essence, nectar. We can accumulate it and distribute it through the senses, between the skin and muscles, into every part of the body. By this kind of relaxation, we can heal even our grasping, shadow side, the unbalanced side that acts against us. The soothing quality of this feeling can heal thoughts, feelings, concepts, and images, embracing them so there is no longer any negative quality.

When we tap and cultivate the source of relaxation and healing energy within our sensations and feelings, we are doing Kum Nye. *Kum* means body, existence, how to become embodied. *Nye* means massage or interaction. In Tibetan, *lu* means our ordinary body; *ku* a higher, more subtle body. In Kum Nye, we activate the *ku*, stimulating feeling, which is *nye*.

When we really *know* how to quicken and develop feelings and subtle energies, cultivating their potential so they feed themselves in an ever-expanding, flowing way, it is even possible to refine, recreate, and regenerate all of the patterns of the living organism. Kum Nye puts us in touch with the pure energies of the body and mind. By increasing our awareness of the immediate feeling-tone of each sensation or emotion, we learn to move within these forms of energy, becoming familiar with different sensory levels, until finally we contact the neutral yet purely wholesome energy that pervades all outer forms.

14

Each Kum Nye exercise has three levels at which the exercise may be experienced, corresponding to three different levels of relaxation. At the first level, feelings have a kind of 'tone' such as joy or sadness, warmth or coolness. These feelings are easy to identify and describe: there is perhaps a tingling sensation, a slightly painful sensation, or a feeling of relaxation and energy flowing through the body. These are 'surface' feelings. We feel them in particular locations in the body, and we remain aware of our 'self' experiencing these feelings during the exercise.

By closely attending to these initial feelings or sensations, we can penetrate to a deeper level of feeling. The first layer of feeling opens to a feeling of greater density and toughness, characterized by a holding quality which blocks energy flow. This feeling cannot be exactly identified, but a 'flavor' remains. Although this layer of feeling is more difficult to deepen than the first, it can be gently melted through a kind of open concentration. At this level there may be a sense of the exercise doing itself, though there is still an awareness of the 'self' feeling the sensation. The self may, however, be experienced as less solid.

At the third level of feeling, we approach pure energy or experience. On this level, all residues of patterning are transcended. There is no longer any feeling that can be separated out and identified, only a kind of melting quality similar to the open-ended quality of extremely joyful feelings. This quality does not seem to reside in any particular location. We do not know where or how it is happening, or what it is; it has no quality of 'whatness'. At this level, the individual ego no longer exists and we become the feeling, merging with it. This is the stage of fruition, the level of completion that is true relaxation.

Once we tap this relaxation, we learn to operate sensations and emotions with a playful, open attitude, and everything becomes relaxation. We know that within every feeling or sensation there is the pure energy— that both 'negative' and 'positive' emotions are flexible manifestations of energy, for only at the surface level do negative and positive, sadness and happiness exist.

Then we know how to use the raw material of experience. At the beginning of any sensation we increase and expand it until it becomes firmly established. When we reach the second layer of feeling we expand that too, experiencing it fully until we pass into the final stage. When the next feeling or sensation arises, we begin again, creating a continuous circle. Then energy constantly refreshes and replenishes itself, and all of the patterns of basic existence, the patterns of our living being, are constantly renewed. Time and age cannot catch and freeze this energy, for it is always actively moving, cultivating itself, never delayed or at a standstill. Sometimes we call this mysterious process 'longevity', and its potential lies within the senses.

Kum Nye practices are like symbols that point to the nature of all existence. By stimulating the very energies of existence, we begin to understand how mind and matter function and interact. We develop an understanding of physical laws—how sensations arise, perceptions develop, concepts come into being, and mental events take place. Aware of the energy and potential in all existence, we learn to see, pursue, and experience this potential. We appreciate the vibrant character of physical form and use this vitality to nourish ourselves. Through feelings, or through the energy embodied in physical form, we learn to experience the physical patterns occurring in our bodies, and understand how matter itself is patterned.

The laws of the universe become transparent. Now we understand that our living organism is no different from a cloud taking shape and dissolving away. We no longer see our bodies as fixed, solid things; we experience ourselves as a process of ongoing embodiment that at any particular moment manifests itself as a physical entity and has the capability to continuously regenerate itself. As soon as we perceive the body not simply as a physical machine but as an embodiment of values and responsiveness, we discover a way of being beyond the usual polarity of 'existence' and 'non-existence'.

When we open to feeling, we no longer see 'energy' only as something that has taken a form with a beginning, middle, and end; we see energy as a whole. It has no limitations, no 'outside'; it carries on the character of numberless forms. Yet the word 'numberless' is not accurate, as the energy itself is whole. Therefore, once we understand ourselves, we can understand others; if we understand our own bodies, we can even understand universes.

When we expand our awareness far enough, we perceive energy as having no subject or object relationship at all. There is only one center, and everything becomes the center. Speaking on the ordinary level we could say that the center is both subject and object, but from another dimension there is no subject-object relationship. The center itself has no limitations or forms; it is a whole. Everything we look at is the center: universe, body, senses.

Preparation

The moment practice begins, you are planting
the seed of a healthy, positive attitude.

Practice of Kum Nye is an exploration and balancing of our inner environment. To benefit most from this experience, the external environment should be made as harmonious as possible. The external environment reflects the internal state of mind, and careful preparation can encourage positive feelings. As experience of the inner world expands through practice of Kum Nye, as you become balanced, appreciation of the external world increases effortlessly. With continuing practice, the separation between external and internal melts away, and you naturally interact harmoniously with our environment.

Choose a clean and quiet place, either indoors or outdoors, where you will not be interrupted or distracted. Complete quiet is not always possible in a noisy modern city, so find as quiet a place and time as possible. Encourage those with whom you live to respect your need for time alone. The temperature should be comfortable, neither too hot nor too cold, and the lighting soft. A carpeted floor or a level grassy place make practice especially pleasant. If you are practicing indoors, you may want to open a window to clear the air, or burn incense. Before you begin, take time to become familiar or reacquainted with your surroundings. Perhaps walk as well as look around; investigate any possible distractions until you feel comfortable turning your attention inward.

During practice, wear loose, comfortable clothing that allows you maximum freedom of movement. As your senses expand, awareness will develop and sensing the texture and weight of materials becomes part of the pleasure of practice. Remove clothes and accessories that might obstruct movement or energy flow, like jewelry, watches, glasses, or contact lenses.

For the sitting exercises you will need a cushion so that your pelvis is higher than your legs. If you find sitting on the ground too difficult, then a straight-backed chair will do. When performing the standing exercises, place your feet on a carpet or the floor, not on a thick mat. For the massage, use a lightly-scented massage cream or a vegetable oil such as safflower or olive. If you use vegetable oil, you may want to add a sweet scent, perhaps musk or cinnamon oil.

Creating an environment conducive to your practice is an expression of a positive attitude toward yourself—even the moment practice begins, you are planting the seed of a healthy, positive attitude. Intrinsic to the practice of these exercises is the decision to find satisfaction within yourself. Nourish this positive attitude and it will grow, developing and increasing your sense of balance, happiness, and relaxation.

All Kum Nye exercises presented here are ways to touch and expand your inner feelings and energies. The external form of the exercises may be stillness, breathing, self-massage, or movement, but the internal exercise or massage, the essence of Kum Nye, is with feeling. From the moment you begin practice, concentrate on the feelings and sensations that arise. Whether you are sitting, standing, or lying down, consider your posture and gestures part of the quality of your experience, and be mindful of how they may affect your feelings. Whenever you move, do so slowly, gracefully and rhythmically.

Just as you cannot truly appreciate the scenery from the windows of a speeding train, when you move too fast in a practice, you will not be able to savor the joy of your discoveries. Every movement can be deeply felt and gracefully performed: imagine the feeling a dancer has when beginning to dance. Execute each single motion with gentle concentration; not a fixated concentration, but a kind of openness that will encourage awareness.

Your experience has an open-ended quality when you learn to practice in this way, for as you perform an exercise, you are aware of the form, texture, and movement of the subtle feelings in your body. Feelings of dullness give way to alert probing and sensing of subtle muscular adjustments and energies; deep insights are then possible.

Participate in each exercise as fully as you can, involving your whole being—your heart, senses, awareness, feelings, and consciousness. Bring all of yourself into the form of the exercise. Let your negative as well as your positive feelings be part of the experience. Kum Nye becomes a dance in which you participate totally. You are not 'working with the body', or 'working with the senses', but fully participating and responding.

Become intimate with your feelings without trying to name or label them. Whenever you feel something, keep the energy of the feeling alive as long as possible, letting it gradually expand and fill you. Broaden your feelings; let them be a mandala, expanding in every direction into time and space. You may find satisfaction in states that are not only within, but are also beyond the senses. Then everything you do can have the quality of these feelings.

The experience of each exercise or massage has characteristics: positive, negative, and neutral. These characteristics are not judgments, for it is as important to feel and work with negativities as it is to work with positive qualities. Awareness of these qualities is an important part of each exercise. Positive feeling is warm and soft and touches your heart. You may experience negative feeling as a dull, dark, heavy sensation in your belly. Neutral feelings are light, balanced, still and calm, part of space.

Taste your experience as fully as you can, chewing, swallowing, digesting, assimilating, and distributing it to your whole body. You will discover different levels of feeling and experience and may become aware of the energy within every molecule and cell. You can increase your awareness and contact with this energy until finally every part of your body acts as a source of energy. When you realize that energy has no location, no 'here' or 'there,' and is abundant and available at any time, then you can truly experience the integration of body and mind.

Approach each exercise openly, without expectation or judgment, for beginning an exercise with expectations of a modality, you cut yourself off from the experience. Judging is one of the obstacles to experiencing. It may sometimes be difficult not to take a critical stance, for most of us judge almost constantly. We may tend to stand outside ourselves, judging our experience and creating an ongoing inner dialogue that occupies and freezes energy: "This feels good," or "I must be doing this wrong."

The key to practicing Kum Nye is to refrain from labeling, manipulating, or trying to make feelings mean something special. When a judgment arises in your mind, use it as a signal to go deeper into sensations and feelings. Observe what organs, tissues, and muscles are awakening; go into these places and explore. Do you feel pain or joy, perhaps warmth or energy? What is the nature of the experience, the tones and qualities?

Although this experience of full participation can be called mindfulness, consciousness, or being aware and sensitive, its nature is unconcerned with naming and defining; there is no longer a critical mind judging. What is happening is what you are doing. There is no need to ask questions or report back to yourself on what is happening. Your feelings simply express themselves.

In learning to relax, we tend to think that there is a goal, and that something must be done to achieve it. The tendency to make an effort is always in the back of our minds, and may become an obstacle to relaxation. Notice whether you come to rely on certain preparations. Try not to arrange anything within yourself—just be natural. There is not any specific thing you must do to relax. When you realize this, you will relax more quickly.

The way to develop relaxation is not to instruct yourself. When you become tied up in plans or explanations, you cannot find internal openness. The secret is just to *be*, without relying on instructions. This may not be easy. We are used to telling ourselves that there is a certain way to be or a certain way to do things. We may even attempt to manipulate ourselves into that mold. When we begin to relax without instructing ourselves there is usually the feeling that we 'do not know how to do it.' As relaxation deepens, however, this feeling of unfamiliarity passes, and there is only allowing and continuing.

In this book you find instructions, including how to sit still, how to breathe, and how to do self-massage and many other exercises. These instructions are important and useful, but when you apply them skillfully, you do not remain caught up in the external description. You move beyond the mechanical level to the level of subtle energy, becoming fully open, without holding back.

Holding back is like continually waiting to be relaxed, expecting relaxation to come from somewhere else. There is a kind of fascinated expectation or inner dialogue— we speculate on success or failure and comment on our 'progress'. In this way it is possible to spend many hours practicing Kum Nye without opening to the energies and relaxation within. So do not let such inner dialogue gain control; relax and let Kum Nye do itself. Direct your energy so that it flows freely—physically, mentally, and emotionally. Be aware and accepting, 'letting go' without seriously paying attention to your inner dialogue or getting involved in it. Simply concern yourself with what is at hand—doing an exercise or massage—and do not worry about results. Then you can develop the open-ended attitude.

During practice, do not be concerned with whether you need more experience or effort to make the exercises work. Simply open the feeling of relaxation as wide as possible. The more you can do this, the fewer distractions, problems, thoughts, and conflicts will arise. The ever increasing experience of relaxation will nurture the body; your whole being will gradually become healthy. There is no need for specific exercises to accomplish this change; your experience of alertness and relaxation is in itself the means to transmute ordinary physical energies. Your body will act by itself.

After completing an exercise or a period of massage, sit and quietly immerse yourself in the sensations. This sitting is also part of the exercise, an opportunity to further develop and expand the feelings that have been stimulated. Warm, glowing, tingling sensations may surface. Stay with the sensations without trying to hold onto them. No effort is needed. Clinging to the feelings, analyzing or categorizing sensations, will interrupt the flow. Remain open, and you find that the energy will stimulate itself.

It will probably take several months before you can truly relax, so it is important to practice regularly. The way to start is to practice Kum Nye for forty-five minutes twice a day, doing sitting, breathing, and movement exercises in the morning, and self-massage in the evening before going to bed. If you wish to spend less time in practice, set aside forty-five minutes once a day. Wait at least an hour after eating before beginning.

Begin slowly and gradually, in a balanced way. There are many exercises presented in this book, but it is wise to limit yourself to three or four for several weeks, until there is an inner awakening to the experience of Kum Nye. Take your time with each exercise. Running from one exercise to the next creates a false sense of progress. True progress does not depend on moving quickly toward more advanced exercises, but on slowly deepening your experience of a single exercise. Spend at least three minutes with each repetition of an exercise, developing your ability to work on a particular experience. Each exercise is a universe in itself and can be fully explored internally.

From time to time, especially in the beginning, you may feel reluctant to practice, as if you are not sure you are willing to relax and feel. Listen to your body to find where you feel reluctant or are holding back, and as you begin Kum Nye, concentrate your energy there. Later, when you have had more experience, you will welcome the sensation of fresh energy in your body.

Your body will naturally seek Kum Nye and, as you practice, it will lead you to the exercises or variations you most need to explore. Sometimes an exercise may happen spontaneously during practice, not because you exert mental or rational control, but because your feelings naturally take the form of the exercise. Once that happens, you develop greater confidence and respect for your body and greater understanding of the nature of embodiment. You are discovering your body of knowledge.

As you explore your body, you will discover sensitive and even painful areas. Breathe into the pain; then exhale slowly and gently and relax the painful area. You will find that with the healing effect of the exercises, pain can be transformed into sweetness.

If a color or image appears during your practice, stop and look for a moment. At times you touch an experience beyond time and space. Energy centers may be opening. As you experience relaxation, the flow of energy within your body may open your heart, dissolving tension there, as well as elsewhere in your body. You will experience an opening of your senses and a heightened sensitivity to taste, color, and sound.

As thoughts slow down, inner harmony will arise. A sense of relief and confidence comes forth. Eventually you will find that feelings of joy, tranquility and harmony expand until you perceive them as expanding out into the universe, and you are aware of nothing else.

Be confident in your Kum Nye practice, and do not give up. Encourage yourself, and patiently go through whatever takes place in the practice. Others, even family and friends, may not support you or even appreciate the value of what you are doing. But your motive in practicing is not merely to benefit yourself. If you want to do your best for future generations of humanity, for your friends and family, you must begin by taking good care of yourself.

This may look selfish, but ultimately our knowledge of ourselves will give us more to share with others. In the beginning we will perhaps give seventy-five percent of out time and energy to ourselves and twenty-five percent to others; later these percentages may be reversed. When we become fully accomplished or enlightened, we can give ourselves fully to others. Then we are free, and everything becomes service.

Sitting

As thoughts slow down, internal harmony arises.
A sense of relief and inner certainty comes forth.

Kum Nye begins simply, with just sitting still and relaxing. Find a place where you can sit on a mat or cushion, or a straight chair. The traditional position for sitting (shown by the Buddha the moment he first became enlightened) facilitates relaxation of both body and mind. Energy flows smoothly in this position, and with enough time, all mental and physical energies become transformed into positive healing sensation. This position has seven 'gestures'.

The first gesture is to sit with the legs crossed. (For these exercises, however, if it is too difficult for you to sit cross-legged, sit in a straight chair with the legs uncrossed. Sit forward on the seat so you do not lean against the back of the chair, separate your legs comfortable distance, and place your feet flat on the floor. This allows the weight of the body to be distributed on a firm triangular base.) When you sit cross-legged, arrange your mat or cushion so your pelvis is higher than your legs. Sitting in the half or full lotus (i.e. with one or both ankles resting on top of the thigh) is helpful but not essential.

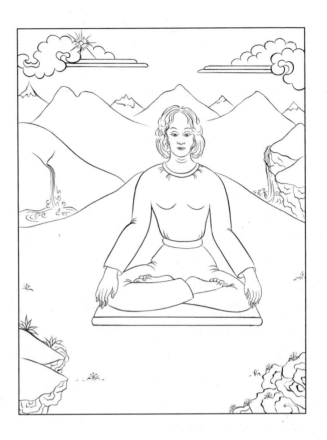

The remaining six gestures are as follows:

The hands are on the knees, palms down. Release tension in your arms and shoulders, and relax your hands so they rest comfortably on your knees. The spine is balanced without being rigid. This allows energy to flow naturally from the lower to the upper body.

The neck is drawn back a tiny bit. Your head will move forward very slightly.

The eyes are half-open and are loosely focused on the ground, following a line downward along the ridge of the nose. Let your eyes be very soft and compassionate, 'Bodhisattva eyes', like a mother looking at her child.

The mouth is slightly open, with the jaw relaxed.

The tip of the tongue is lightly touching the palate ridge, just back of the teeth. The tongue will curve back a little.

As you sit in this way, try to minimize blinking. You can do this by relaxing the area around the eyes and moving your awareness inward.

If you are not used to sitting cross-legged, you may feel some discomfort at first, until you learn to relax unnecessary tension. If you have pain in your knees, cross your legs very loosely and put a higher pillow under your pelvis. The difficulty may be in the knees, but most likely your thigh joints are stiff. The following two exercises will help to loosen the thigh joints. These exercises will be equally beneficial if you are able to sit cross-legged comfortably, but have trouble sitting in the half-lotus or lotus position.

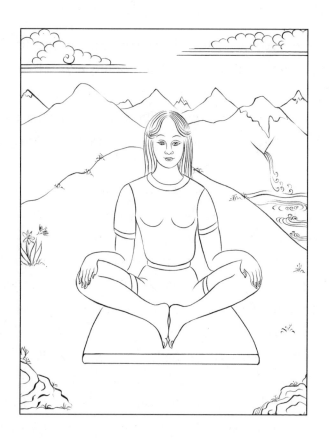

Exercise 1   Letting Go

Sit on a mat or a cushion, with the soles of your feet together, and place the hands on the knees. Bring your feet close to the body. With the hands pushing the knees, begin a light, quick, up-and-down movement in your legs, like the flutter of the wings of a bird. Pay special attention to the upward movement. Continue for about a minute. Then sit quietly for a few minutes, sensing your body. Repeat three times.

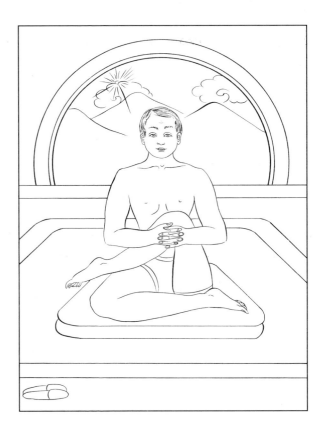

Exercise 2   Melting Tension

Sit on a mat or cushion and cross the legs so your right ankle rests on the left thigh. With your back straight, interlace the fingers and clasp your hands around the right knee. Very slowly lift the right knee a short distance and then lower it. Repeat this three or nine times, very slowly, feeling the sensations in the body.

Then reverse the position of the legs and repeat the movement, three or nine times. When you finish, sit in the sitting posture for at least five minutes, allowing the sensations to continue.

If you need to change position while sitting, straighten one leg in front of you and lift the other knee, placing the sole of the foot on the floor. Clasp the knee of the bent leg with both hands, and sit this position. After a while, reverse the position of the legs. When you feel ready, sit cross-legged again. It is also possible to sit for about ten minutes, massage legs and feet for a few minutes, and sit for ten minutes, continuing for as long as you wish.

Physical discomfort has a mental or emotional component; when the mind is not at ease, the body cannot be relaxed. When uncomfortable while sitting, notice your state of mind. Is there an active flow of thoughts, dialogues, images, and fantasies? In time, you will discover that the sitting posture itself (the seven gestures) and the soft, smooth breathing it facilitates can relieve both mental and emotional agitation and physical tension.

In the beginning, you may think that sitting still means the body does not move; you may hold yourself still. But it is possible to learn to be still without becoming rigid. As you continue to practice, you will discover you do not need to make an effort to relax. Eventually you will experience complete alertness and stillness.

Now sit comfortably in the sitting posture, either cross-legged or on a straight chair. Allow yourself thirty minutes to an hour and try the next two simple exercises.

Exercise 3   Tasting Relaxation

Breathe deeply about ten times, and slowly relax your whole body. Relax your eyes, closing them if you wish, and let your mouth fall open. Let tension slip away from your forehead and scalp. Slowly sense every part of your head—your nose, your ears, your jaw, the inside of your mouth, your cheeks—until the whole head becomes completely relaxed. Then relax the back and sides of the neck, throat, and the underside of the chin. Whenever you find a tense place, enjoy the sensation of tension melting away. Move to the shoulders, chest, arms and hands, the belly, the back, the legs and feet, even the toes. Taste the feeling of relaxation, really feel it, enjoying it more and more until it nurtures every part of your body. Continue for fifteen to thirty minutes.

Exercise 4   Following Sensation

Sit as relaxed and still as you can. Slowly allow yourself to become aware of any sensation or feeling-tone that arises. At the beginning you may have to remind yourself time after time: remember! Follow whatever happens. You may feel a physical sensation or an emotion. The sensation does not need to be strong—it may be light, even delicate.

Be attuned to your inner ear. Trust the presence of your experience and open yourself as fully as you can. Invite the experience in whatever way you do it, without method or formulation. Whenever you feel a sensation or a feeling-tone, allow it to continue and expand as long as possible. Continue for fifteen to thirty minutes.

For the next week, let yourself be as relaxed as possible throughout the day. Relax while eating, shopping, or working. Sensitively watch your movements (even the blinking of the eyes) for subtle patterns of muscle tension. Relax every part of the body, including the breath, the skin, and all the internal organs. Even your hair can be relaxed. Let all aspects of your body have a relaxed, gentle quality. Then you can bring the feelings and sensations alive, and they can inspire and nurture you.

Stimulating feelings and expanding them is the basic activity of Kum Nye. In this way, we learn to increase our enjoyment and appreciation of every aspect of living. Even a minute sensation can be increased, accumulated, and then distributed until it flows throughout the body and expands even beyond us to the surrounding world.

Exercise 5   Expanding Feeling

Sit down very quietly in the sitting posture, and breathe gently and evenly, with your mouth slightly open. Think about some wonderful memory, and let it become very real. Perhaps you remember one of the happiest times in your childhood, or maybe your first love, or a beautiful natural place with fields and a river where you enjoyed to go walking. How do you feel? Create the positive energy of this exquisite memory, expanding it more. Let the body heat up and the breath move a little higher in your chest, until you feel exhilarated. Close your eyes, and increase the feeling of exhilaration until you really feel it bodily.

Expand the sensations with the body, so they become interpenetrating, and you are not sure if they are inside or outside or where their boundaries lie. Keep expanding the feeling, two or three inches outside the body. You are the center of feeling, and from the center the feeling is freely moving out everywhere, in infinite ripples and layers.

Now slowly draw this vital feeling back into the body; you may almost see it physically. Let this energy unite and cleanse the body and mind.

Continue to exercise the exhilarating feeling for fifteen to twenty minutes, first expanding it, creating more and more of the feeling; then bringing it back into your body and senses. If you do this whenever you have beautiful ideas, images, or feelings, your sensory awareness becomes developed in a finer, more substantial way.

Practice this exercise frequently for the next few weeks, daily if possible.

Breathing

Once we know how to contact the energy of breath,
breathing becomes an infinite source of vitalizing energies.

Breathing charts the life rhythms, and the way we breathe signals the disposition of our energies. Agitation and excitement cause the breath to be uneven and rapid. When we are calm and balanced, our breathing is even, slow, and soft. We can change our mental and physical states by changing the way we breathe. Even when very upset, we can calm and balance ourselves by breathing slowly and evenly.

When breathing is consistently calm and even, we will find that energy increases, and health improves. We sleep better and the mental and physical organism become balanced. The mind is lucid, and the body alert and sensitive: hearing becomes clear, colors are vibrant, and it is possible to savor more of the flavors of experience. Feeling tones turn richer, so seemingly insignificant and small things can be enjoyed tremendously, like a little laughter. Once we know how to contact the energy of breath, breathing becomes an infinite source of vitalizing energies.

This gentle breathing links us to a flowing energy or 'breath' that is itself inseparable from the subtle mental and physical energies that move through the body.

This 'energy pattern' is like a mandala, an originating center or zero point from which energy flows in all directions. Within this pattern are energy 'centers' that act as 'terminals' for these energies as they radiate and circulate throughout the body. Among these energy centers are the head center, the throat center, and the heart center. If we could observe this energy pattern from a distance, it would look like a spiral with the head center at the top; seen from above, it would appear as a series of concentric circles with a ring for each of the centers.

The energy of 'breath' is particularly associated with the throat center, which both evokes energy and coordinates the energy flow throughout the body. Therefore, it is through the throat center that we can most easily learn to contact and balance the energy of breath as well as other subtle energies.

The throat center is traditionally pictured as a sixteen-petaled flower with two blossoms, connected back to back. One eight-petaled blossom is directly linked to the head center, the other to the heart center. As energies pass through the throat center they flow outward to these other centers. When the throat center is settled and calm, the energies flow in a balanced and coordinated way: mental and physical energies become integrated, and 'breath' itself is balanced and purified. Usually, however, the throat center is agitated, so these energies become 'blocked,' and do not flow properly.

It is possible, however, to breathe in such a way that the throat center becomes calm and functions smoothly. The way to do this is to breathe slowly and evenly through both nose and mouth, with the mouth slightly open and the tongue lightly touching the palate. In the beginning this is not very comfortable, but as energy begins to travel evenly to the head and to the heart centers, the vitalizing effects of this way of breathing are felt. Then it becomes increasingly easy and pleasant to continue. As the flow of energies within us becomes balanced, our feelings and sensations unfold naturally, and we open to deep sensations of fulfillment.

But this takes time. As the flow of energies throughout our systems is so often imbalanced, we lose touch with our feelings and sensations. This in itself makes it difficult for us to consistently move toward balance within ourselves. Our old habits of reaching out for satisfaction, of looking to others to give us feelings of joy and fulfillment, are hard to break. Yet the more we look outside ourselves for fulfillment, the more we lose touch with our inner sensations. We lose touch with both our physical body and our emotional body.

Once this pattern is in force, it becomes self-perpetuating. Instead of experiencing directly, fully assimilating our sensations and integrating them with the feelings of the heart, we get caught up in patterns of thinking *about* an experience, labeling it and reporting back to ourselves on its nature. We thus reinforce the subject, the 'I,' the one who does the experiencing, and experience itself becomes an object frozen into form and meaning.

When we are in this state, our feelings are actually secondary feelings, interpretations of mental images that we then feed back to ourselves. We live 'in our heads', subsisting on records of past experience, mental verbalizations unconnected to our true feelings. A feeling of continuous dissatisfaction arises, a subtle form of anxiety that we feel in the throat center as a kind of tightness. This tension manifests as the 'self' reaching out for experience. As a result, the flow of energy to the head center increases, and the energy flow to the heart center lessens.

All emotional extremes and imbalances occur in this state: heightened emotion, like anger or hate, as well as severe depression and lack of energy. Until the throat center settles and subtle energies are distributed as much to the heart as to the head, we cannot truly contact the senses or touch our real feelings. Without the energy to activate them, our senses are incapable of operating properly and appear to be asleep.

Kum Nye shows us how to gently dissolve this pattern of anxiety and reaching out, and leads us back to direct experience. By breathing softly through both nose and mouth, we can gradually bring the breath to an even level and balance the throat center so that energies are directed evenly to both the head and heart centers. This steady, even, and yet uncontrolled breathing has an open quality. Even when we first begin to breathe this way, we may feel the senses awaken and begin to stir.

At first, lightly pay attention to breathing equally through both nose and mouth. The quality of the breathing is effortless, without strain. Just let it be natural; you do not need to think about breathing correctly . . . but somehow, way back, your awareness notices that the breath is equally distributed between nose and mouth, and between the inhalation and the exhalation.

As you breathe, your body becomes calm, and you feel relaxed. As soon as you notice the feeling of relaxation, taste and enjoy it. If you do not notice this feeling at first, imagine your ideal of the most heavenly, exquisite feelings. Enjoy them, feel them. Later on you will physically feel the energy. Once you contact the feeling of relaxation, you have found the way. Go into it as deeply as you can; the deeper you go, the richer the feeling becomes, and you can then gather it and bring the harvest to every part of your body. You can feel it in your bone marrow and feel it outside the body as well. Wherever you look, the same feeling is available.

Then just accumulate the quality of that feeling, by stimulating it, making it even richer, deeper, and broader. Encourage the quality of the breath. Let it become exhilarating; accumulate it as water is accumulated to create electrical power. The feeling is joyful, blissful, and open, with a vast merging quality. The feeling becomes so vast that there is an almost overwhelming quality, so powerful you feel you cannot take it anymore. When the feeling builds to this power, it opens all the energy centers, cells, and senses; your whole body becomes balanced.

By steadily practicing this breathing and contacting this feeling, you can accumulate it more and more until finally you directly touch its essence. You need no interpretations or words—you will just be there directly. Then any time you want to use that energy you can. Like adding seasoning to food, you will be able to use as much as you like, whenever you need it.

As you develop the quality of breath, awareness, which arises from direct experience, will gradually expand until breath and awareness become a unity. Then the energies of awareness and breath stimulate each other and energy increases, always fresh and available. The process is like charging a battery: you plug awareness or mental energy into the breath and stimulate energy. This is the secret of abundant energy. Even if your energy is low now, you have lines to it and can reach out for it. When you know how to regenerate your energy and keep it in good supply, you can afford to be generous and give it away, for you have an infinite resource.

When breath is truly balanced—not too controlled or tight, but slow and smooth, at an even level—and when, at the same time, awareness is united with breath as in a marriage, certain effects happens naturally. Breath is like radar, and you are able to sense the signals of any emotion, your own or others. Your awareness of the beginnings of emotion and feeling is like a space that protects you. Awareness becomes an open field, allowing you to exercise awakened control, different from control by suppression or force.

With awareness of the breath, your whole life becomes balanced. Even when you find yourself in situations that arouse great anger, frustration, or pain, you can dissolve the disturbance by just being of aware of your breathing, slightly paying attention and making the breath calm, slow, and rhythmical. The longer you accumulate energy with the breath, the more your whole body calms down; as you give the energy a chance to settle, various parts of the body, at all levels, quiet down. Life has a healthy rhythm, undisturbed by extremes, and the senses can fully ripen and mature.

It is important to work continually with the breath, or else the effects will not last: the body, mind, and senses will slip back into an unbalanced rhythm. So practice this kind of breathing each day for at least three months; twenty to thirty minutes a day is helpful. Try to keep energy flowing, constantly accumulating and generating it with the breath. Start out by being mindful and paying attention to your breathing. Then gradually, day by day, develop a quality of awareness like meditation. It does not matter what you call it—relaxation, awareness, or meditation; these are all just labels. The most important thing is the quality of the experience.

Once we learn to accumulate energy, we can carry on this process day and night, not just at certain set times. The whole body becomes relaxed, muscle blockages dissolve, and energy is distributed everywhere. Our lives become broader and healthier. Later on we may not even have to make any effort at all to tap this energy of breath, for it is behind all physical and mental energies.

External and internal energies both come from the same 'breath' or 'prana', so as our inner landscape changes our relationship with the outside world changes too. The universe becomes much more comfortable to be in. It is as if the outer world of objects and our inner world of the senses—our consciousness—were to merge. We support the world, and it supports us and our senses. Our senses give us pleasure, and we feel positive; we project that, and receive back what we project. Inner and outer become harmonized and balanced.

Begin by breathing very gently and easily. As you progress, breathe more slowly. Just let the breath slow down until it eventually becomes smooth and even, almost without inhalation or exhalation. Your energy will then steadily increase. As you practice Kum Nye check your breathing from time to time to see how you are progressing toward this goal.

Exercises with the Breath

To develop the breathing of Kum Nye—gentle, slow and even, through both nose and mouth—it is best to practice for twenty to thirty minutes every day for at least three months. At first, it may help to separate out the different qualities of breathing. For the first week breathe very softly, as in Exercise 6. For the next three or four days, breathe slowly, as in Exercise 7. If you wish, spend more time on each of these exercises. Then develop an even, balanced breath that is also soft and slow, as in Exercise 8.

In addition, you may want to try some of the other breathing exercises in this section. The sitting position showed in Exercise 10 is a traditional meditation posture. Try it sometimes after massage or exercising. Exercise 12 would best be done in the evening before going to sleep. Exercise 13 is traditionally done on arising in the morning. Exercise 14 is more advanced than the other exercises here, and will be most effective if practiced after a few months' experience of Kum Nye.

Throughout these exercises, let the breathing nourish and relax you, increasing the feelings of enjoyment until they become so substantial they are almost tangible. Let the breath bring more vitality to the body and greater clarity to the mind. Throughout the day, allow the breath to sustain and nurture you. Feel how the senses come alive, giving all of life a magical, spicy flavor.

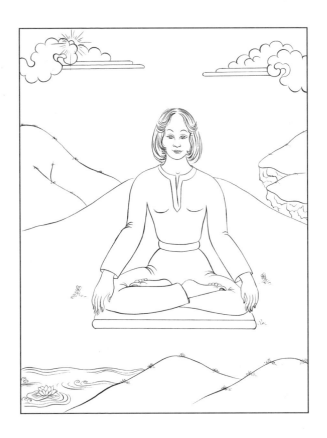

Exercise 6   Joyful Breath

Sit comfortably in the sitting posture (the seven gestures), either on a mat or cushion, or on a straight chair. Make sure your mouth is slightly open, the tip of the tongue lightly touching the palate ridge. Relax your throat, belly, and spine. Begin to breathe softly and easily through both nose and mouth, without paying much attention to the process. This breathing is quite light, yet energizing. When you feel muscle tension, let the breath touch it gently and loosen it.

Bring words and images to the breath and let it soothe and relax them as well. This soft breathing will quiet and settle your whole body. Without trying to control the breath too much, let it gradually become even calmer and softer, until a quality of mellowness develops.

As soon as you feel a sensation—perhaps a feeling of something flowing in your throat and body—accumulate this feeling, not by trying to add anything to it, but simply allowing it to continue. Feel it more. You may feel the sensation moving to different parts of your body.

Practice this breathing for twenty to thirty minutes a day for about a week. As much as you can, become aware of the quality of your breath throughout the entire day. After a week, go on to Exercise 7.

Exercise 7   Opening the Senses

Sit comfortably in the sitting posture (the seven gestures), and begin to breathe softly through both nose and mouth. Lightly pay attention to the inhalation, and gently try to slow it down as much as you can, while keeping the quality of breath as soft as possible. Feel the sensations in and around the body as your inhalation slows down, and enter deeply into them, expanding and accumulating them with the breath. Continue for ten to fifteen minutes.

Lightly pay attention to the exhalation, and exhale slowly through both nose and mouth, keeping the breath light and soft. (As you do this, don't try to do anything special with the inhalation.) As you develop the quality of this slow exhalation, try to open the whole sensory field as much as possible—every cell, tissue, and organ. Let the feelings spread like a halo throughout and around the body. Continue for ten to fifteen minutes.

Practice this slow breathing for twenty to thirty minutes for three or four days. On the third and fourth days, practice twice a day if you can. After increasing the time, pay a little more attention to the quality of your breathing, following the breath with your awareness until you become very still. After the third or fourth day, go on to the next exercise, Exercise 8.

Exercise 8   Living Life in the Breath

Sit comfortably in the sitting posture and breathe softly and slowly through both nose and mouth. Gently pay attention to your breathing so that the breath flows equally through both nose and mouth. Give equal time to inhaling and exhaling.

Notice the quality of your breathing, how sometimes it may be hard and choppy, sometimes agitated or deep. Notice how the different qualities of breathing are related to different mental and feeling states, and how as your breathing becomes easier and more even, the mind settles, and feeling flows.

As you breathe, open the feeling of relaxation as wide as you can. Unite awareness with the breath, and expand any sensations that arise until you no longer know where the boundaries of your body lie; there is only feeling and the subtle energy that rides on the breath.

As breathing becomes more even, you naturally grow more calm. Superfluous muscle tensions wil dissolve, releasing different layers of feeling. As you penetrate to deeper layers of feeling, you will become familiar with subtle feeling-tones, although you may not necessarily have words to describe them. Let the feeling-tones expand so that they become deeper and more vast.

Practice this even breathing for twenty to thirty minutes every day for at least three months. Then continue to practice this breathing whenever you can, when working, walking, talking—during every moment of your daily life, and even during the night, when you awaken.

You may sometimes want to practice this breathing while lying down on your back, either with your legs straight, or with your knees bent and your feet the floor.

In Exercises 9, 10, and 11, a mantric syllable—OM, AH, or HUM—is chanted silently and at the same time unified with the breath. In Exercise 12, the mantra OM AH HUM merges with the breath. You do not need to actually pronounce the sounds; simply be totally aware of them.

The syllable OM symbolizes the energy of existence; AH, of interaction; HUM, of creativity. OM signifies the physical form. AH represents the energy that informs and keeps the physical form alive. HUM points to thoughts, awareness, and activities. Together the mantra OM AH HUM symbolizes the enlightened body, mind, and spirit.

Exercises 9, 10, and 11 can be practiced for either short periods of time, or for long periods such as four or five hours. You may want to begin practicing one of these exercises for a half hour. Once you are familiar with the exercise, try lengthening the time to an hour or more.

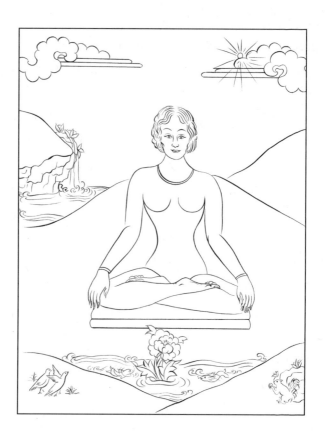

Exercise 9   OM

Sit comfortably in the sitting posture. Breathe gently through both nose and mouth, aware of the syllable OM. Begin to chant OM inwardly, as if on the breath. Let OM and the breath become inseparable. Develop the feeling qualities of breathing OM as fully as possible. You may feel a rising and allowing motion like inhaling, and a gentle, awakened quality to your awareness.

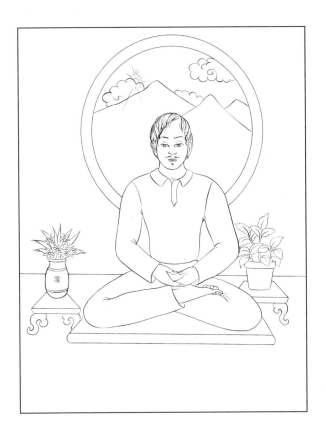

Exercise 10   AH

Sit comfortably. Bring the hands in front of your belly, cradling the fingers of the right hand in the fingers of the left hand, and lifting the thumbs slightly and joining them. Breathe gently through both nose and mouth. Silently chant AH, letting AH and the breath become one. You may feel a silent, concentrated quality, and the breath may become utterly still.

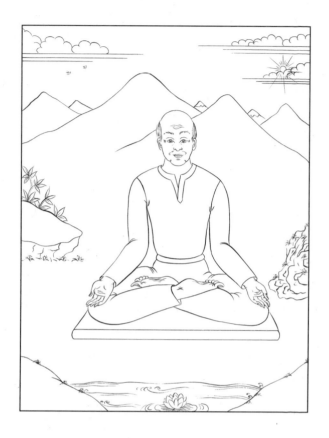

Exercise 11 HUM

Sit cross-legged on a mat or cushion, and place the hands on the knees, with the palms up. Breathe gently through both nose and mouth, and be aware of HUM. Bring HUM into the breath, unifying sound and breath. Develop the feeling quality of this sound and breath as fully as possible. You may feel a subtly sharp, penetrating awareness, a letting go as if exhaling, and a fresh, radiant clarity.

Exercise 12 Breathing OM AH HUM

This exercise is best practiced in the evening before going to sleep. Lie down on your back on the floor with your arms at your sides. Separate the legs about the width of your pelvis. Support the head with a pillow if you are more comfortable that way, and also put a pillow under the knees. Open the mouth slightly and lightly touch the tip of your tongue to the palate. Breathe gently and evenly through both nose and mouth. As you breathe, be aware of the mantra OM AH HUM.

During the inhalation, visualize or think about OM. Hold the inhalation slightly and that becomes AH. When you are ready to exhale, think HUM. Do not actually pronounce the mantra; just be aware of OM AH HUM. Breathe smoothly and casually, giving equal time to inhaling and exhaling. When holding the inhalation, draw in the lower stomach; as you exhale, let the breath go equally from the stomach, nose, and mouth. Breathe a little heavily at the start; gradually and without effort, decrease the amount of air you take in until your breathing becomes very slow and almost silent. At the end of each breath, be still. After a while the breath will continue as if by itself. Gradually shift the focus of your attention from the body to the realm of feeling and energy. It is as if your body expands to a less physical dimension. Continue for half an hour.

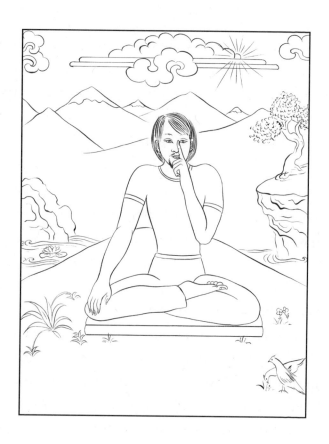

Exercise 13   Cleansing Breath

This breathing is best done immediately on arising in the morning, although it can be done at other times of the day as well. It is meant traditionally to rid the physical system of the impurities that accumulate during the night and to renew the body energies in preparation for the new day. While doing the exercise, imagine blowing out from the left nostril all the attitudes with which you push things away from you, including aversion, dissatisfaction, and fear. Imagine you are blowing out from the right nostril all the attitudes and emotions with which you hold onto things, including desire, attachment, and anger; and imagine that you are blowing out from both nostrils the dull and confused quality of your everyday mind.

Sit cross-legged on a mat or cushion, holding your right hand in the position indicated in the drawing, with the thumb held under curled fingers, and the index finger straight. Rest the left hand lightly on the left knee. Inhale very, very deeply, taking in as much air as possible, filling your belly and chest, and even the spaces at the top of the rib cage. Imagine that this breath fills every cell in your body. Then place the middle joint of your right index finger against the right nostril, closing it tightly. Close your mouth, exhaling slowly through the left nostril as deeply as possible, pushing the very last bit of air out. Keep exhaling until your stomach begins to quake. Then rest for a moment or two, breathing normally through both nostrils. Repeat twice.

Do the exercise three times on the right side, closing the left nostril with the middle joint of the left index finger. Rest briefly after each exhalation. Finally exhale from both nostrils three times as fully as possible. When you think that you have pushed the last bit of breath out, try to expel more. Then sit for a few minutes, breathing normally and enjoying the sensations in your body.

You can visualize the impurities coming out of your body as a dull white stream emerging from the left nostril, a dark red stream from the right nostril, and a deep blue stream emerging from both nostrils.

Exercise 14 Feeling Breath

Sit in the seven gestures. Inhale through both nose and mouth. Hold the breath for one minute, experiencing and expanding the feeling quality. Let your internal rhythm slow down and your senses open. You may feel a rippling or vibrating quality like the energy at the edges of a flame. Whatever feelings and sensations arise, deepen and expand them. Experience them directly, without letting them go into concepts or thoughts or mental images. Then exhale slowly. Repeat the exercise three times.

If you find it difficult to hold the breath for one minute, try holding it as long as possible. As you continue to practice the exercise, you can gradually build up to holding the breath for one whole minute.

Massage

Our feelings and our bodies are like water flowing into water.
We learn to swim within the energies of the senses.

The practice of Kum Nye integrates feelings directly with
the body, instead of channeling them through the mind.
Our feelings and our bodies are like water flowing into
water. First we 'float' in feelings of openness, gentle love
and joy, relaxing and letting the feelings themselves buoy
us up; later there is a lifting feeling of complete confidence.
As we become used to contacting these feelings and the
currents of energy they produce, we learn to swim within
the energies of the senses. A feeling of unity and wholeness arises ... thoughts, senses, mind, and consciousness
join in a kind of inner alchemy. When Kum Nye massage
is done daily for at least six weeks, these feelings become
more and more tangible, occurring not only during practice, but throughout the day.

This internal 'swimming' or massage melts accumulated tension, releasing the energy which has been frozen
at a subtle level by our fixed attitudes and concepts. The
released energy flows into feeling experience, which then
fills every cell in the body. Our bodies become less solid,
more fluid and open, more *ku* than *lu*. As we live and work

59

closer to the energy of feeling and experience, thoughts and feelings merge into one; feelings no longer need to be accompanied by mental commentary. Direct experience is far more substantial and grounded than that channeled through thoughts and imaginings. We grow in awareness.

The immediacy of experience is lost when we allow the minds to grasp at the feelings. So when you begin Kum Nye massage, let go of preconceptions or associations you may have. Thoughts as well as concepts move on a surface layer; as much as you can, go by degrees to a deeper level, the level of experience. Explore each feeling fully. Encourage feelings of joy. Imagine you are in paradise; bring in positive memories, perhaps of beautiful fields, trees, streams, or mountains. Let the feelings express themselves. Happiness is a feeling within your organism that you can stimulate and develop by giving each feeling more flavor, and feeling it as much as you can. Expand each feeling through your senses and thoughts. Thoughts cannot catch you, for you are beyond ego and self-image.

When you continue to deepen and expand a feeling, you will find different feeling-tones that can be explored further. Once you move inside a feeling, it will expand in an inner massage. At first a feeling will bring to mind various images. At a deeper level, the feeling will be deeply nurturing, without images. Finally, you become the feeling, and there is no longer any experiencer or 'I'. Then you are deepening openness, satisfaction, and completion.

Massage means interaction. When you massage yourself, you are not affecting only one place on your body; your whole body participates in the massage. A reciprocal relationship develops between your hand and the muscle or point that the hand massages, generating feelings that stimulate interactions throughout the body. Interaction also occurs between physical and nonphysical levels of existence, and this interaction stimulates certain energies that, not restricted to the body's boundaries, spread to the surrounding world.

When you develop self-massage, you will discover many kinds of sensations and feelings. Kum Nye massage is oriented toward pressure points that stimulate specific energies. You may find that pressure on some places has an immediate effect; pressure on other places may not affect you noticeably in the beginning. Touching particular spots may restore memories or past negativities. As you rub and release pains and knots in your physical body, you may also release mental and emotional blockages.

Muscular patterns related to old injuries may melt down into pure feeling or experience. Pressing certain points may release loving, joyful feelings which open your heart, merging body and mind into one. As your body becomes more fluid and open, you may even discover a time when there is no special purpose to the massage—it is not oriented toward ego or self. Without preparation or goal it just spontaneously happens, is instantly there.

Once the shape of your tension melts down, only feeling or experience is left. Do not label or identify the nature of the feeling, but simply allow it to continue to melt until it flows completely into itself, filling each center, cell, and sense organ with pure energy and experience, like water flowing to the deepest root of a beautiful rose.

As you massage, stretch the bonds of your ordinary conceptions. When you press a certain body point, no part of the body and in fact no part of the universe, need be excluded. Everything can become part of the massage. From a cosmological point of view, absolutely everything participates in the cosmos, and we and the universe are integrated. Our body is a vessel filled and surrounded by space. When we touch our substance, we stimulate ourselves and the universe simultaneously. Our whole body exercises in space.

Massage as Part of Practice

The best way to begin is to massage yourself for forty-five minutes or more every evening for at least six weeks. After six weeks you may continue with the evening massage, or perhaps you will want massage to be a part of your daily Kum Nye yoga practice. Although it is best done in the evening, massage can also be done at other times.

During the massage, wear no clothes or loose-fitting clothes you can easily open, and remove jewelry, glasses, contact lenses, etcetera. Perhaps take a hot shower or bath beforehand; this will help relax tense muscles and open the body to feeling. Use a massage cream or a vegetable oil such as safflower or olive, perhaps with a sweet scent added. After the massage, apply a natural perfume or, if you wish, burn incense. If you are doing the massage right before going to bed, drinking a cup of hot milk with two teaspoons of honey will often help you sleep.

To begin the massage, energize your hands in the way described on page 66. Then slowly oil and rub your body in a random way, without trying to do anything special. Follow your feelings, letting them guide you to where you need especially to rub, and letting them tell you when to increase or decrease pressure. In areas where you feel pain, rub and press with special sensitivity and thoroughness. Let the feelings and the massage move together in rhythm, like music. In this way, slowly massage every part of your body—wherever you can reach. Do not neglect your arms, legs, or feet.

Gradually deepen the experience of the massage, unifying breath, body, senses, and mind. Breathe very slowly and lightly through both nose and mouth; then the breath can awaken and merge with sensation, developing a vital penetrative quality which spreads throughout the body, releasing congested or entangled energies into pure feeling and energy. Expand feeling and sensation to encompass thoughts, so that as you rub and press, your hand becomes the eye of your mind, and your mind enters your body. At the end of the massage, sit still for five or ten minutes and feel the subtle ripples of sensation spreading outward from your body.

After two or three evenings of this sort of 'random' massage, begin to incorporate some of the specific instructions for massage in the pages that follow. Do not rush to try everything, but explore a few new techniques at a time. In the beginning, emphasize your face, head, neck, shoulders, and chest. But as you continue, always feel free to experiment. Find points of stress and blockage and loosen them, slowly freeing the body from its tight inner and outer harness.

Each time you begin Kum Nye massage, awaken the sensitive energies of your hands. Remember that your hand is not a mechanical tool; it is capable of touching your whole body when it appears to touch only a part.

Develop the feelings in the palm, and in each finger and thumb. Whenever possible, use the whole hand while massaging; develop reciprocity between your hand and the part you are massaging, and be aware of subtle linkages to other parts of the body.

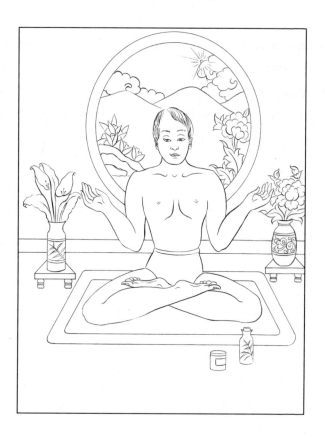

Energizing the Hands

This massage will animate your hands. Do it whenever you begin massage.

Sit comfortably with the back straight, breathing gently through both nose and mouth, and relax. Oil your hands lightly. Bend the arms at the elbows and hold your hands open, with the palms up, at the level of the heart. Cup your hands a little as if holding energy in them. Feel the sensations—perhaps tingling or warmth—in your hands and fingers. Hold the energy in your fingers; then let it pass into your hands like a flame reaching and spreading. From your hands, let the energy pass into your arms, and through your arms into the heart. Allow the whole body to feel deeply nourished by these sensations of energy.

Once you feel these sensations, slowly bring the hands together and rapidly rub the back of the left hand with the palm of your right. You can do this movement quite hard and fast. Follow the sensations—you may feel energy going into the heart and neck and the middle of your back. Reverse the position of the hands, and rub briefly. Now rub your palms together in a rapid motion until they definitely feel hot.

Once again hold your hands open palms up, at the level of your heart, cupping them a little. Take another minute to feel the sensations flowing in hands and body, and then slowly begin the massage.

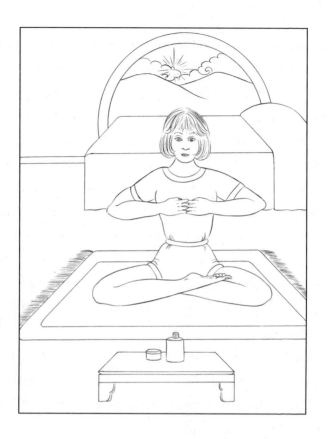

Hand Massage

Massaging your hands with awareness can tune, tone up and enliven the energy of the whole body.

• Interlace the fingers tightly, with the palms and fingers pointing toward you. Pull under tension, massaging down the fingers until they spring apart in release. Repeat the pulling and massaging, and feel the sensations awakened in your body by this exercise.

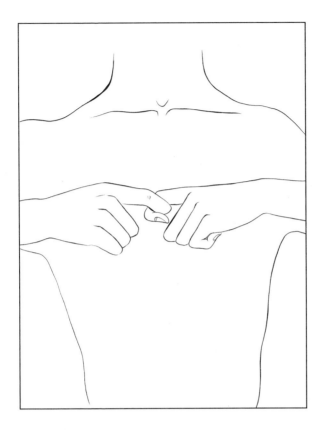

• Hook each finger separately with the corresponding finger of the opposite hand. Pull under tension until the two fingers gradually slip apart.

• Massage each fingertip on one hand with the fingertips of the other hand.

• Massage down each finger from the fingertip to the base. Move slowly, making sure to work the sides as well as the front and back of each finger.

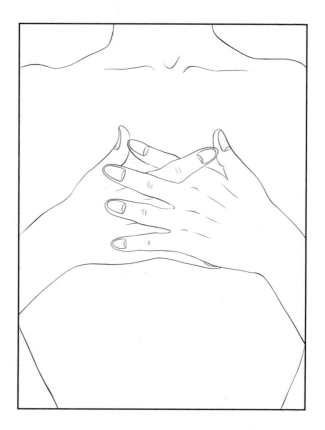

• Place the base of the finger to be massaged in the 'web' between the index and middle finger of the other hand, and grasp the finger firmly. Slowly pull the finger while twisting it gently, moving from the base of the finger to its tip.

• Work on the back of your hand between each of the small bones, the metacarpals, massaging in the direction of your fingers. Give particular attention to the large area between the forefinger and the thumb.

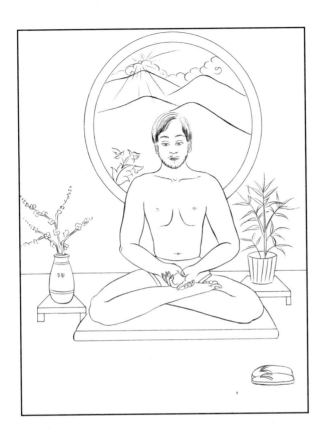

• Massage the palm of your hand with the thumb of the other hand. You can also use the larger knuckle of the forefinger to move across the palm. Deeply massage the large mound of the thumb as well as the smaller mounds below the fingers. Massage between each finger. Pay attention to all of the small muscles between the bones, tracing them from the heel of the hand to the fingers. As you massage, breathe softly and evenly through both nose and mouth.

The next part of the hand massage uses pressure points. As you press these points (and later when you press points on other parts of your body), be aware of the effects that are produced by different degrees of pressure. At first press lightly; gradually develop medium pressure; when appropriate, press strongly. When you want to diminish the pressure, do so gradually: first subtly lighten the strong pressure, then reduce it to medium, and then slowly to light pressure. In this way you develop awareness of six distinct stages of the massage. With more practice, you may develop additional subtleties of pressure.

Be careful not to release pressure too suddenly. This 'shocks' the system and loses the subtle qualities of feeling. Experience fully the lifting up and putting down of your hand and fingers. When you remove your hand from your body at the end of the massage, do so almost imperceptibly; then the feelings will continue for quite a long time.

• The hands have many sensitive and powerful points that can stimulate interactions throughout the body. To find the first point, turn your hand palm up and look at the 'rings' at the inside of the wrist. Place your forefinger in the middle of the ring nearest the palm. Then turn the palm down and place your thumb on the second point, which is on the back of the hand exactly opposite the first point. Hold your wrist tightly between your thumb and forefinger, and press strongly. Relax your chest and belly and other places where you have unnecessary tension; breathe gently through nose and mouth.

Now reverse the position of thumb and forefinger, placing your forefinger on the back of your hand and the thumb on the inside of the wrist. Strongly press and manipulate the two points simultaneously. Release the pressure gradually, sensing the feelings that arise.

Keeping the thumb on the same point on the inside of the wrist, move your forefinger about a finger-width down towards the fingers and to the side nearest your little finger. This point (point 3 in Figure 1, page 74), between the bones of the little finger and the fourth finger, may be sensitive. Once you have found this place, exert strong pressure with both thumb and forefinger and hold. Release slowly and gently.

Now move your forefinger to the corresponding point on the side of your hand nearest the thumb (point 4 in Figure 1). It is approximately one finger-width down and to the side of the second point. Again press strongly with both thumb and forefinger and hold. You may feel strong sensations, even pain. Stay with the feelings, breathing through nose and mouth. Release the pressure gradually.

Now turn your hand palm up. Measure two finger-widths down (toward the fingers) from the first point to the fifth point, and place your thumb there. Then place your forefinger on the point on the back of your hand exactly opposite this point (point 6). Strongly press these two points simultaneously. Release slowly, breathing gently and evenly through nose and mouth.

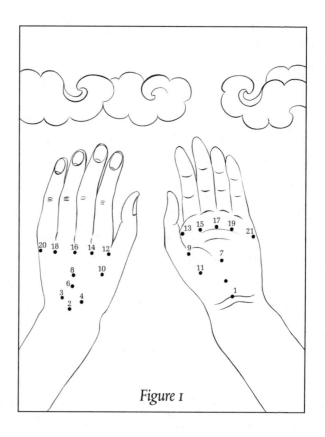

Figure 1

Place your thumb on the point in the middle of your palm (point 7). Place your forefinger on the corresponding point on the back of the hand, between the bones of the middle and fourth fingers (point 8). Press these two points simultaneously in a sensitive way, gradually increasing the pressure. Release slowly.

Now place your thumb on the point near the thumb webbing (point 9). Place your forefinger on the opposing point on the back of the hand (point 10). Now press these two points simultaneously, sensitively increasing and decreasing the pressure. Remember to breathe gently through both nose and mouth.

Now place your thumb on the point in the middle of the thumb mound and press and rub sensitively (point 11). The pressure can be strong.

The remaining ten hand points (points 12–21) form a row across the knuckles. There are five on the palm and five on the back of the hand. Two pairs of points are at the sides of the hand, and three pairs are between the knuckle-bones. Work these points in pairs, placing your thumb on each palm point and your forefinger on the corresponding point on the back of the hand. Gradually increase and decrease the pressure.

Complete the entire massage, including the pressure points, on both hands.

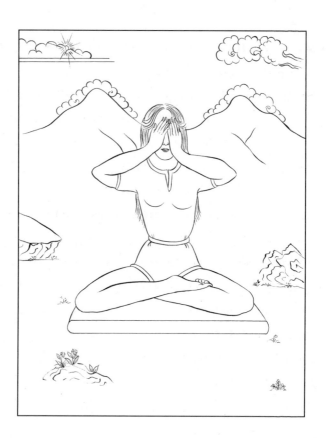

Face Massage

Our heads are usually busier than the rest of the body, and emotions—that are closely connected to thoughts—tend to constrict our facial muscles as well as our necks and shoulders. As you massage your face, feel the energy move throughout your body.

• Energize your hands in the way described on page 66. Once your palms feel hot, slowly bring them up to your face and place them gently over your closed eyes, without any pressure on the eyeballs, and without touching your nose. Your fingers will overlap a little. Leave your hands in this position for several minutes, sensing the movement of heat and energy into your eyes. Notice connections with other parts of your body; you may feel heat penetrate through the eyeball into many body parts.

Again rub your palms together. When they feel hot, place one hand on your forehead and the other on your chin. Close your eyes and feel the energy flow. Repeat, reversing the position of your hands.

• Massage around the orbit of your eyes, touching each point firmly and gently. Massage both eyes at the same time. Begin at the inner upper edge of the eyesocket, and use your thumbs to find a notch in the bone just under the eyebrow (points 1 in Figure 2, page 78). Press up, gradually increasing the pressure, and hold. Keep your head erect. Close your eyes and go into the feelings; they may be quite powerful. Release the pressure very gradually, and stay with the feelings which are produced.

With your first or middle finger, trace under the upper ridge a short distance from the first point to the next small valley or notch (points 2 in Figure 2), and press and massage it gently. You may want to close your eyes as you do this. Trace under the upper ridge to the third small valley or notch, near the eyebrow's arch. Spend extra time here,

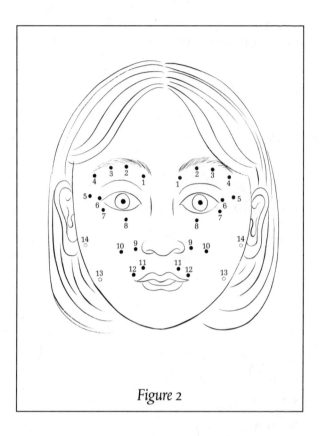

Figure 2

pressing and massaging gently with your first or middle finger. Experiment with different degrees of pressure.

At the upper outside corner of the eyesocket there is another place that deserves special attention (points 4). Use the tip of your first or middle finger to locate and massage this small crater in the bone.

Follow the curve of the eyesocket down to a little bump in the bone, a finger-width from the corner of the eye (points 5). Press with your forefingers, increasing and decreasing the pressure.

78

Use your forefinger to move just inside the corner of the eyesocket to the sixth point. Press gently breathing softly through both nose and mouth.

Trace with your forefingers a short distance to the seventh point, just inside the eyesocket, a little below the sixth point. Press gently.

Follow the lower curve of the eyesocket to a notch in the bone below the center of the eye (points 8). Press gently and delicately. Give particular care to the area where the lower eyesocket meets the bone of the nose.

• Hold your eyebrows between thumb and forefinger, at the inner edge. Press your thumbs up a little so they rest against the bone and give support from below. Lightly squeeze the eyebrow between thumb and forefinger, and rub slowly back and forth with the forefinger. Work out to the outer edge of the eyebrow; then return to the inner edge and repeat the massage.

• With your middle fingers, press and rub the place where you feel a deep depression in the temples. Rub very slowly in a circular motion. When you find a sensitive spot, move even more slowly. Press very lightly at first, and gradually increase the pressure. Be sure to release the pressure very slowly. Then change the direction of the circles and continue to massage, letting your feelings guide your rhythm and pressure.

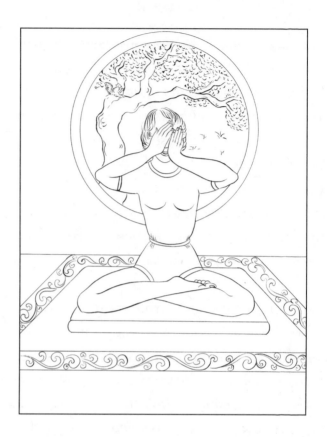

• To massage your forehead, place the fingers of both hands side by side on the left side of the forehead. Slowly draw your hands horizontally across your forehead, bringing as much of your hand in contact with your forehead as you can. Move slowly back and forth several times.

• Now massage down the sides of your nose. Begin with your forefingers on each side of the nose near the corners of the eyes, rubbing slowly and thoroughly with an up-and-down motion. You can use two fingers or even all your fingers, although the forefingers are enough for the job. Move slowly down the sides of your nose, varying the pressure. Give special attention to the areas where the bone of your nose ends, about halfway down your nose, where your nose flanges meet your cheek, and below your nose, where your teeth begin (see points 11 in Figure 2 on page 78).

At these places press your fingers in deeper and then rub slowly back and forth. Pay attention to any special feelings that may be released. When you finish rubbing at the base of your teeth, begin to move upward again. Do this complete movement two or three times.

• Place your thumbs at the corner where your nose flanges meet your cheek. Your hands will hang down in front of your chin. While pressing your thumbs into this corner, slowly rotate your hands until your fingers point toward the ceiling.

Pressing strongly up under the cheekbones, rub your thumbs back and forth across the area just below the cheekbones, out to the side of your face. The movement of your thumbs is quite subtle although the pressure is strong. Follow the line of the cheekbone up to the bony ridge near the ear. Let your sensations expand, releasing subtle tensions under the skin.

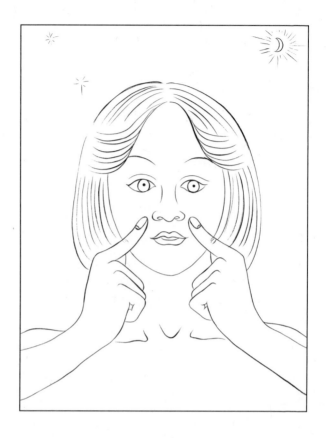

• With your forefingers, press points 9, on either side of the nose (see Figure 2 on page 78). As you gradually increase the pressure, breathe evenly through both nose and mouth and allow your sensations to expand. Do not hesitate to develop strong pressure.

Then follow the line of the cheekbone away from the nose to points 10, just past the curve. Again, press strongly, gradually increasing and decreasing the pressure.

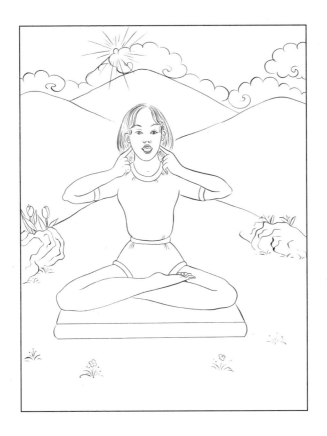

• Slowly massage across your cheek to the point just on the corner of the jawbone (points 13 in Figure 2). Press gently here with your forefingers, yawn a little, and slowly move your elbows out to the sides, so your chest feels as if it is opening. Do not press heavily on this point. Continue to press, yawn, and open your chest a little more. Relax your belly and keep your breath slow and gentle. Then slowly let your elbows come forward, and release the pressure.

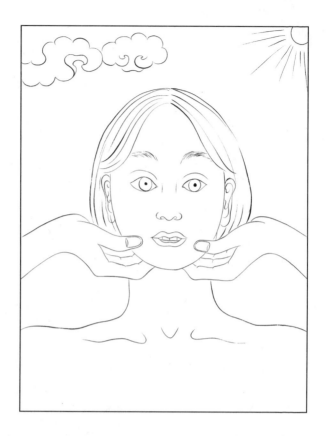

• Now place your fingers under your jaw and rest your thumbs on the chin, as shown in the drawing. Both the elbows are pointing out to the sides. Using all your fingers at once, press up under the jawbone and work very thoroughly along the whole line of the jaw. Do not be afraid to press strongly and remember to release the pressure slowly. You will also be able to press along the top of the jawbone with your thumbs. Breathe gently through nose and mouth as you press.

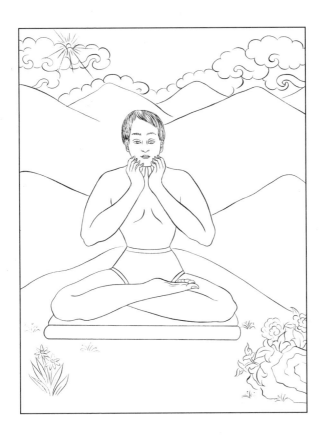

• Place your thumbs under your jaws, near the throat, resting your fingers on your chin. Open your mouth slightly, and gently press your thumbs up under the jaw. Manipulate this whole area with your thumbs, pushing up, especially near the root of the tongue and tonsils. This area may feel thick and gunky; notice if you feel reluctant to touch it. Create a dialogue between your thumbs and these neglected muscles and see if you can bring this area alive. Relax into whatever feelings come up as you press. The musculature of the jaw holds tight habit patterns of thought and behavior, and massage here may release a variety of feelings. With your hands in the same position as above, use your fingers to massage along the upper line of the jaw.

• Smile, and manipulate the corners of your smile with your thumbs. You will discover habitual muscle tightenings which you can relieve with this massage.

As you rub, you may also be able to massage the gum and the base of some upper teeth through your flesh. When you finish rubbing, slowly relieve the pressure. How does your face feel?

• At this point in the massage, when you have covered all of the major areas of the face, it is especially pleasurable to massage the whole face in a slightly different way.

Massage up the center of the forehead and across the forehead to the temple area. Then massage from the bridge of your nose across the cheeks toward the ear.

Massage across your face from the area under the nose to the ear.

Massage around the mouth, feeling the bone structure underneath your skin. Press points 11 and 12 as shown in Figure 2 with your forefingers.

Massage across your face from the mouth, deeply manipulating the chewing muscle. Massage along the edge of the chin to the angle the jaw.

• Place one hand across your forehead and the other directly above it on your head, the fingers of each hand pointing in opposite directions. Simultaneously move both hands slowly in the directions the fingers point; then slowly move them back. Continue rubbing, moving the hands down your face to your chin, then back up again to your forehead. Let the hands contact your face as much as possible. Try this massage after taking a shower.

• This massage is for both face and head. Place hand across your forehead and the other hand across the back of the head. (Be sure to remove glasses and jewelry.) Slowly move your hands in opposite directions, one hand across your face, the other across the back of your head; then move them back. You may feel as though your hands are rotating your head, although your head is motionless during the massage. Continue, slowly lowering your hands until you massage your whole head. Continue past your chin to the throat and the back of the neck. Enjoy the full contact between hand and head.

• Use your thumbs and forefingers to massage your ears. Start at the outer edge of the ears and work toward the center in a spiral movement. Manipulate and massage each tiny section, breathing softly and evenly through both nose and mouth, merging breath and feeling. If your ears become hot, gently stop.

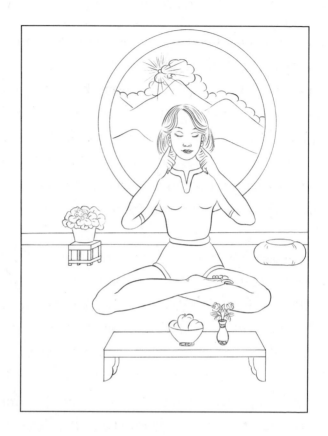

• Just behind the earlobe there is a small crevice. Close your eyes, and with your forefingers, press and rub near the top of the crevice, carefully and sensitively, without much pressure (points 14 in Figure 2, page 78). You may feel a connection with your nostrils. Close your mouth and continue to rub very slowly and not too strongly while inhaling through the nose only. Bring whatever sensations you feel into the massage. As you continue to press and rub, inhale a little more through the nose, flaring your nostrils, and relaxing your lower body. Keep your back straight. Then rub more and more slowly, feeling the sensations in your body, until finally you stop rubbing.

Now place your thumbs on this point, press lightly and with your forefingers slowly rub your temples in circles, first in one direction, and then in the other. Breathe softly and evenly through both nose and mouth, and as you rub, let the breath accumulate sensation and distribute it to every cell of your face, head, and body.

• Massage your face with special attention to what is bone and to what is not.

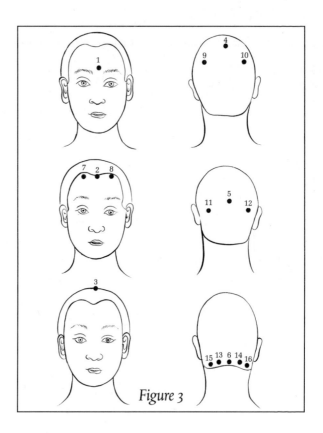

Figure 3

Head Massage

Usually we are more aware of our faces than of the rest of our heads. But the head has sensitive areas and points which can relieve subtle blockages throughout the body, gently awakening the senses.

• Massage your scalp with all your fingertips. Separate your fingers and place the fingertips firmly on the front of the scalp with the thumbs on the sides the skull.

Keeping the fingertips in place, massage back and forth so that the scalp moves across the skull. Try this massage at different tempos. Touch every part of your scalp, moving from the front to the center of the back of your head.

• Starting at the top of your head, trace the muscles down the left side of the back of your scalp to the neck, using all of the fingers of your left hand. Then use your right hand on the right side of the scalp, keeping your head straight. Spend extra time at places of pain or pleasure.

• The rest of the head massage deals with a group of sixteen pressure points (see Figure 3). Points 1–6 are on a midline over the top of the head, running from front to back. Points 7–16 are found to the sides of points 2, 4, 5, and 6. With a few exceptions, the points are four finger-widths apart.

Gently explore these points until you become familiar with the feelings they stimulate. Do not neglect the side-points. As you rub and press them, breathe slowly and evenly through both nose and mouth, unifying breath and sensation. Go deeply into the feelings stimulated at each point, paying particular attention to the variations in sensation that are produced by different degrees of pressure. Especially as you slowly release the pressure, sense the subtle, flavors of feelings that develop.

Once you are familiar with the points, you may want to develop the longer massages such as those for points 3 and 6.

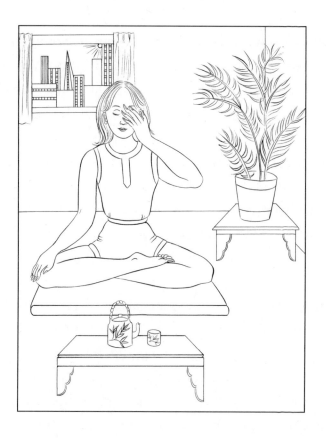

Point 1: To find this point, commonly called the 'third eye', measure four finger-widths up from the tip of your nose. To do this, place the fingers of your right hand on the nose so that the little finger rests on the tip and the forefinger is near the eyebrows. Keep the fingers together and straight. The point is just beyond the forefinger. When you put pressure on this point you may feel a slight depression and a special sensitivity that indicates the right spot.

Place your middle finger on this point and rub straight up about an inch and then down again, exerting some pressure. Close your eyes and look inside in a relaxed way, concentrating on the point. With eyes closed you feel more as you rub, and the feelings are more likely to continue when you cease rubbing. Breathe through nose and mouth. When you sense a kind of energy, transmit layers of this feeling to the center of the body. Once you feel the energy there, slowly distribute the feeling from the center outward to your whole body, letting it become part of every muscle. After a few minutes, let the rubbing subside, and sit quietly with your hands on your knees, continuing to sense the feelings that have been produced.

Tension is closely related to the process by which the mind produces images. Rubbing this place relieves much of that tension and stimulates the senses so feelings begin to spread throughout the body like an inner halo. Body awareness and mental awareness merge, united with the breath.

As this relaxation deepens, the ideas and images we produce become more balanced and vital, and of more benefit to others. Our bodies and minds are so richly nourished and sustained from within, and we are able to be truly caring to everyone. We can benefit from each moment's precious opportunity to expand and share the joy of being alive: as joyful feelings spread to others, they become more balanced as well.

Pressing the next group of points will help to release muscle tension throughout the body.

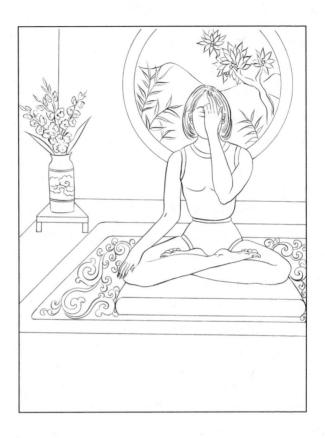

Point 2, 7 and 8: Measure four finger-widths from point 1 to point 2. With the first and middle fingers of one hand, press this point, and without lifting up, massage one inch above the point and then down again. Repeat several times. Massage points 7 and 8, which are an inch to each side of point 2, using both forefingers. Then again massage point 2. Alternate pressure on point 2 and points 7 and 8 for several minutes.

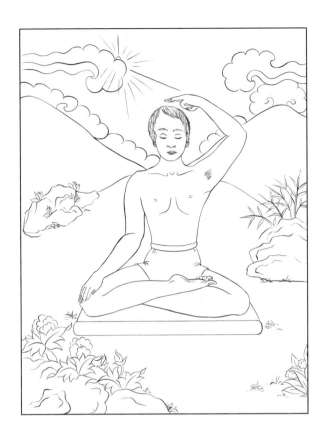

Point 3: Measure four finger-widths from point 2 to point 3. This special place is the healing center of the body; it is also the gate through which consciousness passes when we die. Through massage and visualization, we can gently open this center and learn to heal ourselves.

• With three fingers, draw a circle at this point, rubbing and pressing lightly. As you rub, visualize a circle two inches in diameter. Close your eyes and lift your fingers up, touching your hair softly. Raise your fingers higher, two or three inches above this point, and then lower them, without hurrying. Continue to lift and lower the fingers until you feel something, perhaps an open or cool feeling.

Do not be concerned if at first you feel nothing special. It may take a while. Just continue to concentrate loosely on this point while sensing with your fingers. Later it may be possible to feel a little energy there when rubbing with only one fingertip.

• Once you are able to visualize a circular opening on the top of your head, visualize the extension of this circle into an open column from the top of your head to the base of your torso. Spend four or five one-hour sessions if you want to develop this visualization.

• When you are able to clearly visualize the open column within your body, visualize sparkling white universal energy pouring into it. This beautiful white energy slowly fills the column, flowing down into your throat, heart, and navel areas, reaching to the very root of your body. The energy is inexhaustible; you can hardly imagine it. It comes from all directions at once, moving like a spiral around a core.

When you practice this visualization for forty-five minutes each day during one week, you may feel the special joyful quality of this healing energy. If you do not contact this feeling at first, try to imagine it, and in time you will feel it. When you do, you no longer see your body; there is only the beautiful white energy filling the open column like milk in a pure crystal glass. Each cell and molecule takes in this healing energy until it is completely saturated.

Points 4, 9, and 10: Measure four finger-widths from the middle of point 3 to 4. From the fourth point measure four finger-widths down on each side of the head (see Figure 3). Again, a special feeling, almost of pain, indicates the right places. Concentrate on the side-points rather than on the fourth point itself.

Close your eyes, and rub and press point 9 with the left thumb and forefinger, and point 10 with the right thumb and forefinger. Whatever you feel, let yourself become that feeling, and go with it wherever it goes. Release the pressure gradually, breathing evenly through both nose and mouth, allowing the sensations to spread and be distributed throughout the body.

Hold the scalp muscle tightly between thumb and forefinger and rub up an inch and down an inch from the middle of each point. Rubbing these points vigorously will loosen tension in the neck muscles.

Points 5, 11, and 12: Measure four finger-widths from point 4 to point 5; from the fifth, measure four finger-widths down on each side to locate the two side-points (see Figure 3). Focus on the two side-points. With eyes closed, rub these two points slowly with your middle fingers, breathing softly through both nose and mouth. As you rub and press, bring breath, mind, fingers, and sensation so close together that you are no longer sure if you are being massaged by hand, mind, feeling, or breath. Let your awareness and your breath enrich your sensations until they become so full and open-ended they spread beyond your body, stimulating nurturing interactions in the world around you.

Point 6: This is the most important of the points. It is located at the back of the neck near the juncture of the skull and the spine, approximately four finger-widths from the center of the fifth point. It may be a little difficult to find at first—it is not in the same place on everyone. If you cannot find it the first time, you will find it another, particularly if you work regularly with the pressure points on your head and face.

You can approach this point by gently rocking your head back and forth, with eyes closed. Support your forehead with one hand, and with two or three fingers of the other hand press at the back of your neck near the base of the skull. The spot you are looking for can be anywhere within two or three inches of the top of the spine. Perhaps you will find an edge or corner that will lead you to a very sensitive area. You may feel a tiny cracking inside. There

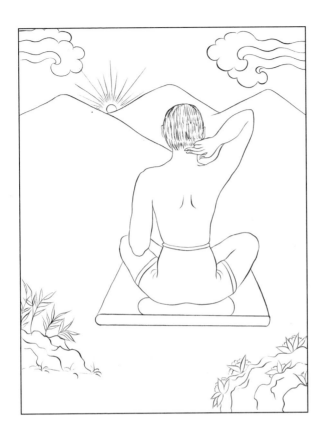

is special energy at this point, a deep kind of pain that is easily transformed into pleasure. Sometimes it seems like a delicious feeling. When the rubbing produces a special or strange feeling, you have found the right place.

Expand this feeling as much as you can. Inhale a little more deeply and let the exhalation flow gently. Discontinue rocking your head, but continue to manipulate the point; work with it as if it had four corners, each of which you press and rub. Relax the stomach and let your body be still and calm. Imagine that you are flying like a bird and that your body is light and airy. Go deeply into the feeling. Sometimes this feeling can be so deep and sensitive that you feel you want to cry. Distribute the feeling all the way down the spine to the sacrum.

This feeling brings all the subtle senses alive. Many tensions become caught in this place, and rubbing it refreshes all bodily energies. Feeling washes through the spine and the backs of the shoulders, sometimes reaching the heart.

Points 1 and 6: Simultaneously rub and press the first and sixth points, concentrating lightly on the sixth. It does not matter if you cannot find the exact place of point 6. Even if the two points are not connected in a direct line, simultaneously pressing those two areas stimulates a special energy which relieves various sensitive blockages.

Close your eyes, and rub the two points strongly with equal pressure for about thirty seconds. Then release the pressure slowly, sit very still, and concentrate loosely on the back of your head and neck. Feel the energies moving through your forehead, perhaps above the eyeballs, to the back of your head and spine. If you do not feel anything, tighten the eyeballs a little, keeping your eyes closed. Then slowly loosen them, and notice any sensations in the back of the neck or head. Perhaps there is a sensation of heat, or a warm and blissful feeling. Sometimes you can almost feel the neck muscles becoming warm and light. There is a gentle quality to this warmth, like touching the body of a tiny new baby. Feel it more, concentrating loosely on the back of your neck and sensing the feelings flowing down your spine and perhaps into your heart.

If you want to develop this particular massage, practice it for forty-five minutes a day for at least two weeks. If possible, practice twice a day.

Points 13 and 14: These points are approximately one inch to each side of the sixth point, along the base of the skull. Use your middle fingers and gradually develop strong pressure as you rub these points.

Points 15 and 16: These points are approximately one inch from points 13 and 14, toward the ear and down a little, near the tip of the mastoid process. Use your middle fingers to experiment with different degrees of pressure on these points.

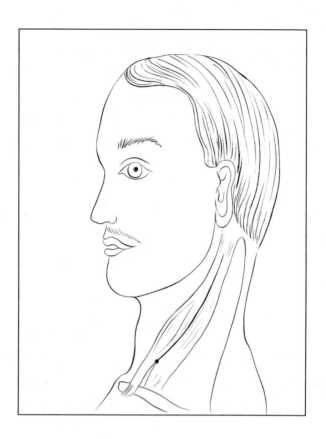

Neck Massage

As your neck becomes more relaxed, your head and heart become integrated, and your feeling capacity grows.

• With your middle fingers, find the bumps in the skull just behind your ears and begin to stroke down the neck muscle. (Use your left hand on the left side, and your right hand on the right side.) You may want to use two fingers. Stroke, rub, and also press down this muscle, the sterno-mastoid, following it down the neck to the shoulder. Then return to the bump behind the ear and repeat.

Near the shoulder, the muscle separates into two strands. See if you can feel this slight separation, and as you massage, try to widen it a little. Press the point where the muscle separates with your middle fingers, gradually increasing and decreasing the pressure. Continue massaging this muscle for at least ten minutes. Also try massaging the muscle on the left side of your neck with your right hand; then use your left hand on the right side of your neck. Explore different degrees of pressure, remembering always to release the pressure very slowly.

• Press the sterno-mastoid muscle between your thumb and four fingers, working up and down the muscle in this way. Then clasp your hands behind your neck and knead this muscle with the heels of your palms. Breathe softly and evenly through both nose and mouth as you massage, and bring your awareness to the breath. Let the gentle influence of the breath permeate the tensions in your muscles and mind, releasing nurturing feelings.

• Using the first and middle fingers of the left hand, knead, press, and stroke down the muscles along the left side of the back of your neck. Repeat on the right side with the right hand. Let relaxation expand, unifying body awareness, mental awareness, and breath awareness.

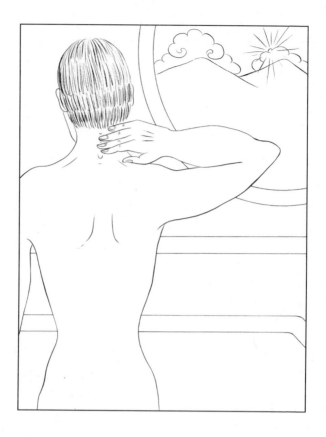

• With the index or middle finger of one hand, press just above the large vertebra at the base of the neck. (There is a large bump there on a line with the shoulders.) Slowly move your head back and then press the point strongly. Your finger should be able to go in quite deeply. Release the pressure gradually.

Then slowly move your head forward and again press the point strongly. Release the pressure gradually, breathing gently through nose and mouth. Very carefully lift your head.

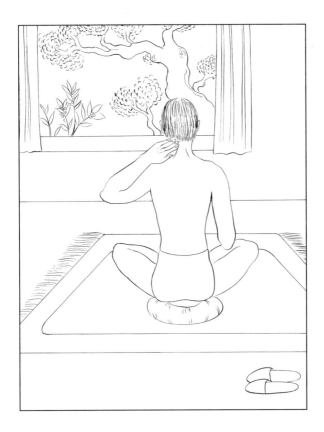

• Massage the left side of the back of your neck with your left hand, stroking in from the sides toward the center-back of your neck in a slightly upward direction. Then repeat on the right side with your right hand. Keep your head up and your chin in as you do this.

• This is a turning movement from the front to the back of the neck. Place the right hand under your chin with the heel of the hand near the hollow of the throat, the fingers and thumb all curving around the right side of the neck.

Keep your chin up. Slowly glide the right hand around to the right and slightly up to the center-back of your neck. Your whole palm and all your fingers touch your neck; thumb and fingers are together.

As your right hand moves around the neck, place the left hand under your chin, thumb and fingers together pointing to the right, and slowly follow the path of the right hand. As you complete the turning movement with the left hand, begin again with the right. Continue to develop the movement until it becomes smooth. Change the position of your hands and in the same way massage the left side of the neck.

• Bend your head so your right ear moves toward your right shoulder. Pass first your left hand, fingers pointing up, and then your right hand up the left side of the neck along a line from the base of your throat just above the breast bone, to the area just behind the ear, and then along the base of the skull to the center of the back of your head. You will be following the contours of the sterno-cleido-mastoid muscle. Continue this massage for several minutes, developing a smooth and steady stroking motion with your hands.

As you stroke, breathe gently and evenly through both nose and mouth. Let the breath melt the outlines of hand and neck, merging them together. Gently end the stroke; then bend your head toward your left shoulder and continue the massage on the right side of your neck.

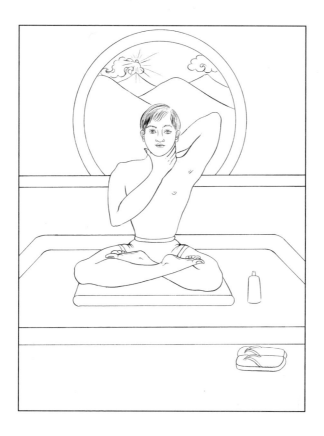

• In this stroke, you alternate between massaging your throat and the back of your neck. Encircle the base of the throat with your right hand, thumb and fingers on either side of the throat. Hold the throat firmly, almost tightly. Place the left hand on the back of your neck, thumb and fingers together, the heel of your hand on the left side of the neck and your fingers curved around to the right side.

Begin the massage by stroking up the throat with your right hand, opening your mouth slightly as you stroke. Use your full hand for this massage, all of the palm and fingers touching the skin. Stroke up your throat and up under your chin—lifting the chin as you stroke under it—until your hand moves off the edge of the jaw bone. As you do this, support the head with your left hand.

Then return the right hand to the base of your throat, and support your head from the front as you begin to stroke up the back of your neck with your left hand. Your head will bend forward as you stroke. Continue just past the base of the skull, then return your left hand to the base of your neck and begin again to stroke up your throat with the right hand. Let the massage be very soft, gentle, and calm, and allow yourself to feel the sensations generated throughout your whole body as you apply pressure. Do the complete stroke at least three times.

• Place the hands at the back of your neck along the base of the skull with the fingers pointing toward each other. Move across the muscles, stroking out from the spine to the sides of your neck. Use the thumbs as well as the fingers. Press strongly as you stroke.

When you reach the sides, bring your hands back to the spine and repeat the movement, a little lower than the first time. By the third time, you will have moved crosswise over the full length of your neck. Continue the massage for several minutes, breathing gently through both nose and mouth, expanding your feelings and sensations. Relax your belly and the area around the eyes.

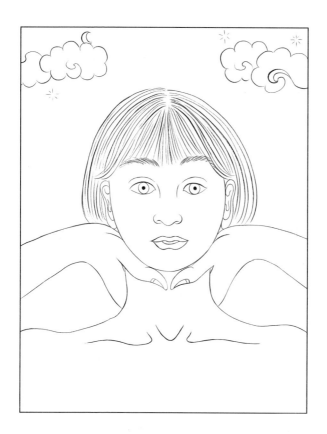

• Place both hands around your neck with the thumbs under the chin and your fingers at the back of your neck. Slowly stroke down the length of the neck, with as complete contact between your hands and your neck as possible. Continue at least a minute.

• Place your right hand under your chin, with the thumb and middle finger on the muscles on either side of your throat and the rest of your hand in as much contact with your neck as possible. Open your mouth slightly, and lift your chin a little. Stroke down the neck, beginning with the left hand as soon as there is room under the chin. Stroke down the front of your neck with one hand following the other closely, so that the second stroke begins before the first one ends. Continue, alternating hands, for several minutes, breathing gently and evenly through both nose and mouth.

You may want to do the neck massage, or portions of the massage, at various times throughout the day—whenever you feel tense. Difficult situations and problems always seem to catch us when there is the least time to deal with them. Tension builds up, often settling in the neck, as well as in the musculature where the neck meets the shoulders and the head.

When you are feeling especially tense, notice if you are holding tension in the neck. Although you may feel as if you have no time to spare, relax for a few minutes. Slowly begin to rub your neck. You may wish to rub very lightly at first. Lightly concentrate on soothing feelings spreading from your neck down your spine, into all your limbs. Let warm, nurturing sensations spread up into your head as well. These feelings will lighten your whole body and heal tension in the mind, so that you think more clearly. When the mind and body are relaxed, both work better; problems take care of themselves and the days become lighter and easier.

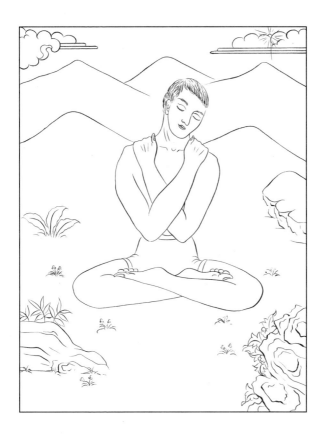

Shoulder Massage

Our shoulders are often tense with unexpressed feelings. When we gently release these tensions, feeling flows more smoothly between the chest and neck, and between the front and back of the body.

If you are pregnant or have had a neck injury, omit the head rotation in this massage.

Cross your arms and rest your hands on the opposite shoulder, close to your neck. Keeping your hands in this position, use your middle fingers to massage the shoulder muscle in a circular movement (see Figure 9 on page 147). Move the fingers slowly, pressing strongly. As you do this, rotate your head clockwise, with eyes closed. Coordinate the two movements. After three clockwise rotations, make three counter clockwise rotations. Remember to move very slowly and to breathe gently and evenly through both nose and mouth. Release the pressure slowly as the rotations come to an end. Sit quietly for a few minutes.

• Press with the middle and index fingers of one hand on the back of the opposite shoulder near the arm, where the bone of the shoulder blade divides (see Figure 9). As you press, slowly rotate your shoulder first in one direction, then the other, gently breathing through nose and mouth. Increase and decrease the pressure gradually. Repeat the massage on the other shoulder.

• In whatever way seems best to you, massage the shoulders, working over the top of the shoulder and down the shoulder blades, moving toward the spine. Then work back up to the top of the shoulder, using pinching and rotating movements. The powerful trapezius muscle which covers the shoulder and upper back holds many tensions, even pain; work with knots and tender areas until they become relaxed. Spend at least ten minutes on this massage.

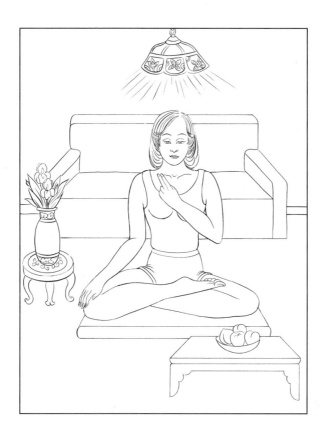

Chest Massage

Massaging the chest will improve breathing and energy circulation, and opens your heart to feeling. Especially women have a tendency to hold tension in this area.

• Using one or two fingers, press along the collarbone from the base of your neck out to your shoulder. Then press along and between each rib of the chest from the breastbone to the side of your chest and where possible,

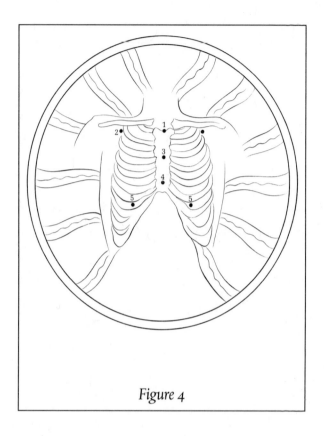

Figure 4

under your arm. There are many sensitive points located along these paths. Work thoroughly, in a meditative way, breathing into the area you are massaging.

Be certain to pay particular attention to points 1–5 in Figure 4. (Point 1 is located just above the breastbone; point 4 is the midpoint between the nipples; and point 3 is midway between points 1 and 4.)

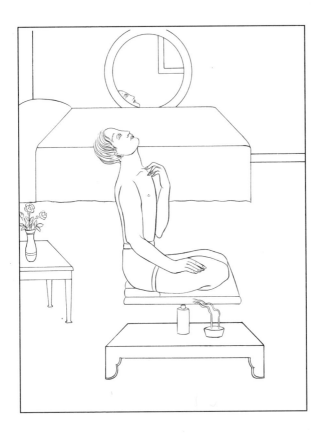

• Press the point just above the breastbone (point 1 in
Figure 4) with your index finger or thumb. As you do so,
gently yet firmly, arch your spine and neck backward, but
do it with care, and without straining. Do not let your head
go all the way back.

Hold the posture for a minute, continuing to press
strongly. Breathe gently and evenly through both nose
and mouth. Then very slowly release the pressure on the
breastbone, and straighten your spine and neck.

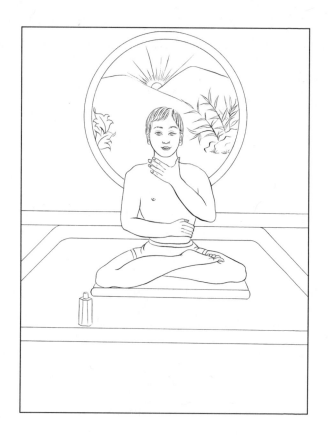

• This massage is for both the chest and the belly. Place your left hand at the base of your throat, the thumb and fingers on either side of the throat, and place your right hand on the left side of your waist. Make sure both hands are in full contact with your body. Very slowly and firmly, simultaneously glide your left hand down over your chest and belly to your left waist, and your right hand up your belly and chest to the base of your neck. Your hands will move along parallel paths, in opposite directions. Then in the same way, without stopping, move your right hand down to the left side of your waist as you move your left hand up to the base of your throat. Continue this massage for several minutes, developing a steady rhythm, paying attention to feelings that arise. Join your feelings to the breath; then bring them into the massage and let them deepen the quality of the rhythm.

End the stroke in a gentle way; then place your right hand at the base of the throat, and your left hand on the right side of your waist. Continue the massage for several minutes on the right side of your body.

• Place your right hand near the top of the left shoulder and your left hand near the top of your right shoulder. Keeping both palms in contact with your chest at all times, move the two hands toward each other and then away from each other. Move them rhythmically back and forth until you have covered the entire surface of your chest. Continue slowly for at least one minute, breathing through both nose and mouth.

• Place your hands flat on the sides of your body, as close under your armpits as you possibly can, with the fingers pointing downward. This may be a little difficult at first. Pressing firmly, slowly move your hands down your sides to the hips. Let the contact between hands and body be as full as possible. Breathe softly through both nose and mouth. Continue for several minutes.

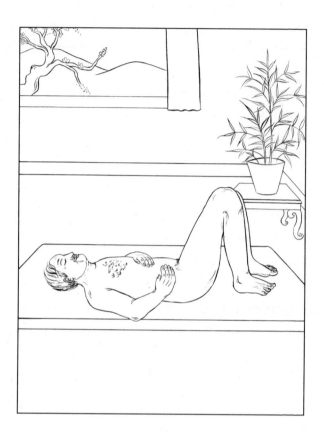

Belly Massage

When the belly truly relaxes, we become free from grasping. Massage here is especially important for men, since it is common for men to hold tension here.

• This massage is best done in the evening, at least one hour after eating, and without clothes. Lie on your back with your eyes closed. Separate your legs a comfortable distance, bend your knees and draw your feet toward your body a little. Relax your belly. Place the right hand on your lower abdomen and the left on your upper abdomen. Let the contact between your hands and your belly be as full as possible. Slowly begin to massage in a large circle, moving your right hand up on the right side of your belly and your left hand down on the left side. When the left hand crosses over the right arm, let hand and arm touch each other as completely as possible.

At first massage with light pressure; gradually develop medium and finally strong pressure. Press especially deeply on the left side. Then decrease the pressure, passing gradually through each stage until the pressure is so light you are not sure your hand is touching your belly at all. Take at least five minutes for this massage. This motion follows the curvature of the large intestine.

• Gradually move one hand to the upper border of your belly and the other to the lower border, near the pubic bone. Place the edges of your hands against your body, so the palms face each other. Hold your breath a little, but not too intensely.

Without hurrying, push down with the upper hand and up with the lower hand, making your belly into a ball. Be entirely relaxed in the upper part of the body, especially the chest and neck. Remember to hold the breath. Exhale slowly, then repeat several times.

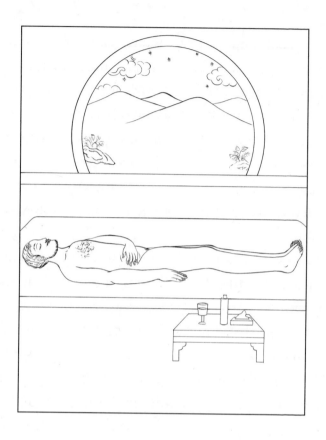

• Place your left hand on your belly, with the fingers point-ing to the right. Push your belly out a little and keep it there, breathing gently through nose and mouth. With your hand in place, develop a slow circular movement with the edge of the hand and tips of the fingers, pressing deeply into the belly, especially on the left side. Continue for several minutes, creating a steady rhythm and joining the rhythm to the breath.

• Now in any way that feels appropriate to you continue to massage the superficial musculature of the belly area. Massage up on the right side of your abdomen, across the area under the ribs to the left, and down on the left side. Then massage more deeply, kneading all the internal organs and tissues, starting under the ribs and working down into the pelvic area. Again, work down on the left side and up on the right. When you find a tense place, spend more time there. Breathe easily, and let the breath soften and melt the edges of your tension. Allow the breath to pass into the very center of the tension, carrying soothing feelings which will calm and nurture you.

When you feel ready to stop, repetition of the first stroke in this section—simultaneous circling movements with both hands—will let you come to a natural conclusion. Then lie quietly for a few minutes, breathing gently.

When you are away from home, perhaps in a tense or emotional situation that is giving you difficulty, the belly massage can be particularly helpful. It produces feelings of relaxation that flow outward from the belly, affecting your whole outlook, enabling you to think clearly and act effectively. What appeared to be unpleasant may even become enjoyable. You can do the belly massage even when it is not convenient to lie down. In a sitting position, support your lower back with one hand and rub the belly with the other hand. When you rub in circles, be sure to rub up on the right and down on the left.

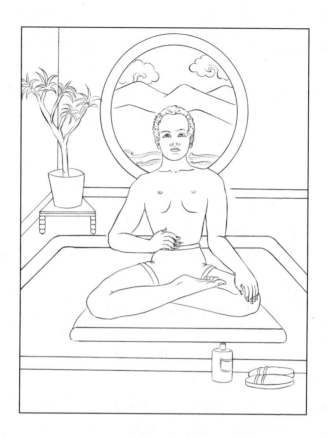

• You can do the following massage in a sitting position: strongly press the navel (there is a pressure point in that area) with the middle finger of one hand while arching your spine and neck backward. Be sure to not let your head go all the way back. Rest the other hand on your knee. Hold for a minute, breathing gently through nose and mouth. Then slowly straighten your spine while gradually decreasing the pressure. Explore the feelings generated by the massage.

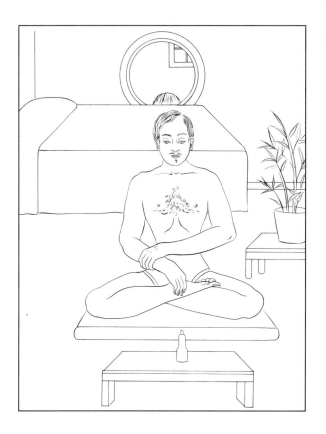

Arm Massage

Massaging the arms improves both breathing and circulation so they become rhythmic and balanced. Muscles throughout the body are strengthened, and a fresh pure quality is stimulated within the subtle energies.

• Massage your forearm in rings the width of your hand. To do this, grasp your left wrist with the right hand so that thumb and middle finger meet at the inside of the wrist.

Slowly turn your right hand in one direction until you have made as complete a ring as possible. Squeeze and press the arm as you turn your hand. Then shift your hand up your arm one hand-width and turn the hand in the other direction to make the second ring. By the fourth ring you will be up to or a little beyond the elbow.

• The rest of the forearm massage is oriented to the pressure points illustrated in Figure 5. Massaging these points will generate many flavors of feeling.

To find the first point, bend your left arm at the elbow so your hand points to the ceiling. On the back of your upper arm, measure the width of three fingers up from the point of the elbow in the direction of the armpit. Press strongly on this point with your right forefinger. Straighten your neck a little as you press. Then slowly stretch out your left arm in front of you, palm up, and continue to press and manipulate this point. Take time to experience what you feel. Then slowly work down the length of the back of the arm to the wrist, as if drawing a straight line from this point. Slowly rub and press as you move down the arm. When you feel a little pain or find a sensitive spot, spend more time there. You may eventually be able to locate specific nerves in your arm.

Find the first point again, and from there measure approximately two finger-widths to the left and two finger-widths to the right. Here are the next two points. Point 2 is toward the inside of the arm; point 3 is toward

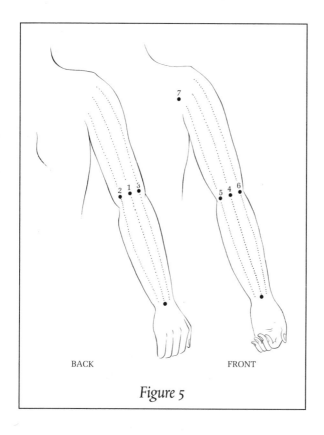

BACK   FRONT

Figure 5

the outside of the arm. Both points are located on the back of the upper arm. Once you have found these points, mentally divide the back of your arm into three sections lengthwise, picturing a line from each point running from behind the elbow lo the back of the wrist. Straighten the arm and begin to press the second point steadily. Slowly develop more pressure; finally, press strongly. Release the pressure gradually. Work your way down the imagined line to your wrist and back up to the second point. Repeat the same sequence for the third point.

• There are also three pressure points on the front of the forearm which can be followed down to the wrist. To find the fourth point, straighten the arm with the palm up and press the middle of the crease or ring at the inside of the elbow. Use one or two fingers. Press very strongly. Then, without releasing the pressure, move down an imagined line to the inside of your wrist. Exert steady pressure. Give special attention to the point at the wrist (this is point 1 in Figure 1, page 74). Work slowly back up to the fourth point.

The fifth point is approximately two finger-widths from the fourth point toward the inside of the arm. If you do not find it exactly there, bend your arm at the elbow and place a finger where the elbow-crease ends, on the inside of the arm. Then straighten the arm and exert pressure at this point with one or two fingers. This point may be a little painful. Press deeply into the muscle. Then work down the imagined line to the wrist. Press rather strongly, allowing the sensations you feel to expand. Throughout the massage breathe gently and easily through both nose and mouth. Slowly work back up to the fifth point.

The sixth point is about two finger-widths from the first point, toward the outside of the arm. This point may be the most sensitive of the three. Press the point, rubbing forward and back and to the sides. Pay attention to the quality of the feelings generated. Rubbing here may release sensations in the heart area, the neck, and the intestines. Slowly work down the imagined line to the wrist. When you reach the wrist, go a little beyond the farthest wrist-crease. There is a special place next to the bone. Press this point with your fingers, one at a time, keeping the arm almost straight. Then massage back up to the sixth point, being especially aware of any sensations in your heart area. Be sure to do the complete forearm massage on both of your arms.

• Now massage the upper arm in rings from elbow to shoulder, as in the first forearm massage above.

Massage from each of the three pressure points on the back of the arm up to the top of the shoulder and down again to the elbow. Do the same for the three pressure points on the front of the arm.

Massage the deltoid muscle over the shoulder cap and the biceps muscle on the front of the upper arm until they have no knots or sore areas in them. These muscles both tend to become overdeveloped in men. There should be a continuous flow from one muscle to the next, yet each individual muscle should be able to move alone.

Rest your hand on your knee, and straighten your arm as you gently massage the biceps with the other hand. Straightening the arm will help to increase the length and freedom of the biceps. Be sure to do the complete upper arm massage on both arms.

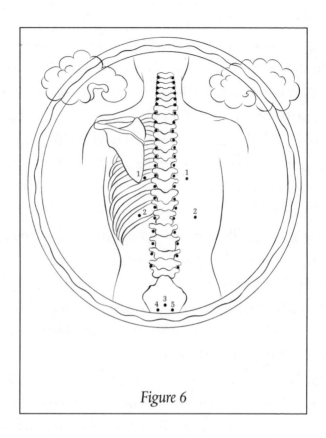

Figure 6

Back Massage

Massaging the back helps to release feelings of joy and love and gives life and strength to all the senses.

• Start at the side of your chest, in the armpit, and massage toward the center of the back. Take your time and massage the large muscles in this area thoroughly. Work around and on top of the shoulder blades. Do first one side of the back, then the other.

128

• There are two pressure points just above the lower curve of the shoulder blades (points 1 in Figure 6). Press these points with your middle fingers, at the same time or separately. Experiment, slowly increasing and decreasing the pressure.

• Points 2 in Figure 6 are on the muscle at about the level of the kidneys, exactly opposite chest points 5 (see Figure 4, page 114). Press both of these back points with your middle fingers, gradually developing strong pressure. Release slowly. Then use one middle finger to press one back point and the other to press the corresponding chest point. Go deeply into the sensations stimulated by this pressure. Then repeat with the other pair of points.

• With your both thumbs, press the three points on the sacrum (points 3, 4, and 5 in Figure 6), gradually increasing and decreasing the pressure. Using the thumbs wherever possible—and the middle fingers when the thumbs cannot reach—strongly press between the vertebrae, working from the base of the spine up to the base of the skull.

• Lie on your back on a mat or soft rug. Separate the legs a comfortable distance, bend the knees, and place the feet flat on the floor. Raise your pelvis up from the floor, shifting your weight toward your shoulders. With both hands massage around the sides of your body toward the back.

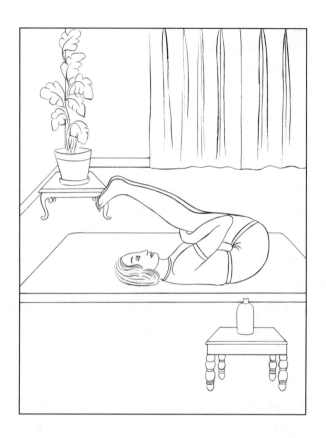

• The following backward roll will massage the upper area of your back where your hands cannot reach. Sit with your legs a comfortable distance apart, your knees bent and your feet flat on the floor. Hold your left knee with your left hand and your right knee with your right hand. Without moving your legs, slowly lean backward until your arms become straight and the small of your back is as close as possible to the floor. Then draw your feet along the floor toward you and roll backward, straightening the legs. Roll forward to return to the sitting position.

Be sure the small of the back touches the floor during the roll. Repeat several times.

• Roll backward in the manner described above, and stay on your back. Draw the knees close to the chest. Put your arms around the knees, and roll from side to side a little, massaging your back as fully as possible. Roll gently for a short distance, but not so far that you lose your balance.

This massage and the backward roll massage will relieve tension throughout the length of the spine. As the muscles alongside the spine relax and lengthen, sensations of well-being and joy are released. Nurture yourself with these feelings; let them touch you inside the heart. While doing these massages, move so gently and softly that your body loses a sense of definite form: you become part of the feeling of joy. Your sensation is not captured in just one corner of your body; it spreads to every part. This sensation can become so large and full that it extends beyond your body, and you become part of a universal sensation. The boundaries between you and the world around you dissolve.

• Now lie on your stomach and massage the sides of your body and your back, moving your hands toward the center of your back. It feels good to use the knuckles in this area.

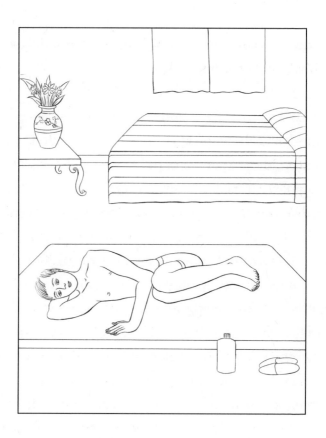

Hip Massage

Massaging the hip helps to stimulate feelings and energies that become blocked from lack of exercise.

• Lie down on the floor on your right side with your legs fairly straight, your left leg in front of the right. Start at the waist, and use both hands to massage the left hip and buttock in the direction of the leg. Try massaging with your fists as well. Small circular movements with the knuckles will help to loosen tension. If you discover any sensitive areas, massage thoroughly there, merging the breath with your sensations and opening the feeling of relaxation as wide as you can. If you do not feel much sensation at first, simply continue to bring your breath and your awareness into the massage; then sensation can awaken within you. Continue with the next part of this massage before massaging your right side.

• Tuck one arm under your head as a pillow, and place the other hand flat on the ground near your chest. Straighten your legs and rest your left leg on lop of your right. Slowly lift both legs six inches or so above the ground. Without lowering your legs, bend your knees, pressing the calves as close to the thighs as you can. Hold briefly, and then bring your knees close to your chest. Be aware of the pressure of your right hip against the floor. Now straighten your legs, lowering them gently to the floor, and rest. Repeat slowly two times.

Explore the feelings generated by the massage. Feel the flow of energy from the hip to the legs and feet; then feel the flow of sensation to the upper part of your body as well. Instead of feeling the sensations in your hip, feel the sensations in the rest of your body. By massaging your hip you can spread healing and invigorating feelings throughout your whole system. Now roll onto your left side and repeat the two parts of this massage on the right side.

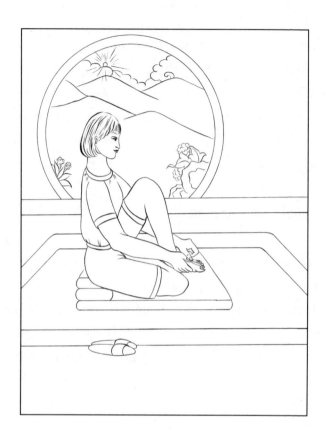

Leg Massage

Lack of exercise prevents the flow of feeling in our legs as well as our hips, and massage here can begin to awaken sleeping energies. When you exercise regularly, massaging the legs sensitively can eventually smooth the flow of sensation, relieving subtle blockages.

• Sit on a mat or cushion with your left knee bent and your left foot flat on the floor. Rub between the big toe

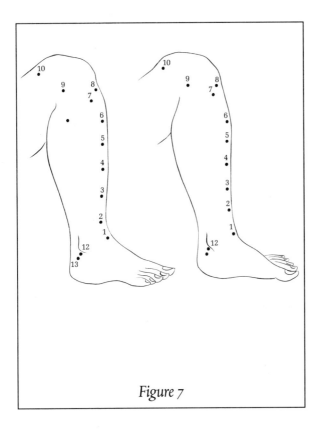

Figure 7

and the second toe, tracing between the tendons up to the ankle. Continue stroking up the shinbone to the knee, with thumb and forefinger on either side of the bone. Massage especially the pressure points 1–6 along here, as indicated in Figure 7. Should you find clusters of tension or pain, return at intervals to rub them in small circles until any knots loosen and perhaps dissolve. Breathe gently through both nose and mouth as you rub. Repeat the massage for the right leg.

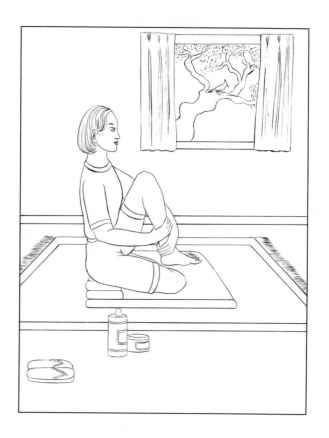

• With both hands grasp your leg just above the ankle, one hand above the other, thumbs at the back of
the leg. Simultaneously twist and press both hands
right, then left, as you work up the shin to the kneecap.
Hold your leg firmly as you twist, letting the contact
between hands and leg be as complete as possible.

Change the position of your hands so the thumbs are
on the front of the shin, and repeat the leg twist.

• Massage your knee, the four corners of your kneecap,

at the sides of the knee, and behind the knee. Using your thumbs, press the four sets of points (points 7–10) on and around the knee at the locations pictured in Figure 7. If you do not find these points at first, do not give up; you will find them as you go deeper into feelings and let them guide you. Breathe evenly through nose and mouth as you explore with your fingers. When you find a point, experiment with degrees of pressure; release the pressure slowly.

• Press strongly with the thumb on the point approximately five and a half inches down from the top of the kneecap on the outside of the leg. Release the pressure slowly.

• To massage the thigh muscles, place one hand on the back and one hand on the front of the thigh. Rub from side to side in large, sweeping movements, pressing as strongly as you can. Make certain your whole palm is in contact with the leg as you rub. Move your hands in the same direction; then move them in opposite directions. Then place one hand on the inside and one hand on the outside of the thigh and continue the movements. Also explore for any knots or painful places by tracing the muscles up from the knee area with your fingers. Give a circular rub with four fingers to any tense places you find. Pay special attention to the places where the thigh muscles join the hip and knee.

Now reverse the position of your legs and repeat the leg massage for the right leg.

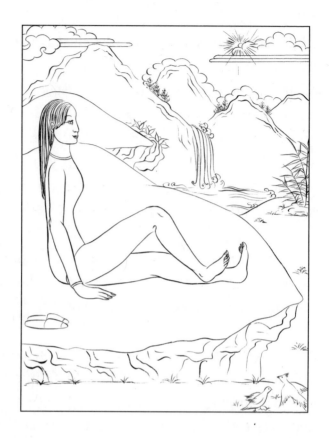

• Sit with your legs outstretched in front of you, and lightly place your palms flat on the floor near your hips. Relax your legs as much as you can. Bend your right knee, and place the pad of the foot high up on the left leg, near the groin. Use the right leg and foot to massage the left leg, curling around it and moving up and down its entire length and around the sides. Continue for a few minutes. Then change the position of the legs and use the left leg to massage the right.

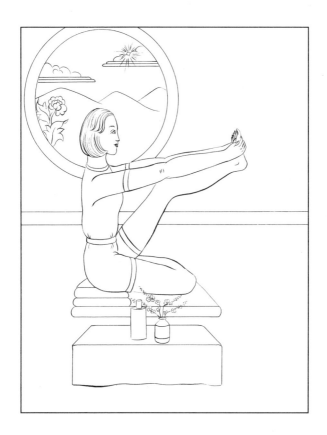

Foot Massage

Like massaging the hands, massaging the feet can tune and vitalize the whole body.

• Sit on a mat or cushion with your back straight and your legs loosely crossed, the left leg outside the right. Lift your left knee, interlace your fingers, and use them to support the ball of your left foot. Push your foot against your hands, straightening the leg in front of you as much as possible.

Feel the stretch in your leg and the ball of your foot and hold briefly. Then slowly lower the leg to the floor. Repeat for the right leg and foot.

• Cross the left leg over the right, resting the left shin on the right thigh. Support the foot with your right hand on the heel and grasp the toes in your left hand. Vigorously rotate the toes in a circle, first in one direction and then the other. Then extend the circles so you are rotating the ball of the foot as well as the toes. The whole upper part of the foot can participate in these widening circles. Vary the rhythm, rotating alternately slowly and quickly.

• Still grasping all the toes with the left hand, bend them back and forth several times. Then extend the motion so the ball of the foot as well as the toes bends back and forth. The foot is very relaxed during this movement.

• Massage the toes of the left foot, using the fingers of both hands. Apply pressure to the pads of the toes. Then massage each toe, one at a time, from the base of the toe to the pad. Be sure to massage the sides as well as the front and back of each toe. Direct pressure as well as rotating motions may be used. Pull gently on each toe to stretch it.

• Massage the areas where the toes join the sole, using the thumb or knuckle. Press the four pairs of points between

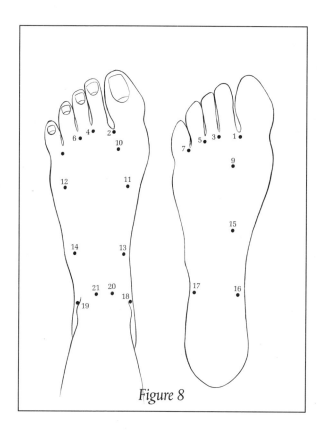

Figure 8

the bones pictured in Figure 8 (points 1–8). Use the thumb on the sole, and the middle finger on the top of the foot.

• Move to the ball of the foot; using the thumbs of both hands, strongly probe each joint. Press deeply between the pads of the ball of the foot. There is no danger of harming yourself, so do not hesitate to press as hard as you like.

When you find a sensitive place, trace it briefly, and try to become acquainted with it. Touching certain sensitive places may release memories.

• Give special attention to point 9 in the pad of the foot immediately behind the bulge of the big toe. Release the pressure very slowly. With your thumb on point 9, place the forefinger on point 10 on the top of the foot and work these two points simultaneously.

• With the thumbs on the ball of the foot, use the fingers to press the top of the foot. Then move the thumbs to the instep and continue rotating pressure on all parts of the top of the foot. Include points 11, 12, 13, and 14.

• Now return to the sole of the foot. Use the knuckles and the fist of the right hand to exert rather firm pressure all over the sole of the foot. Include point 15, in the middle of the sole.

• With the thumbs, stroke the length of the sole diagonally, starting just in front of the heel on the inside of the foot. Alternate your thumbs, creating a continuous sweeping rhythm. It is important not to break the contact between hand and foot during this part of the massage. Then stroke diagonally from the side of the foot, near the heel, to the ball of the big toe. You may sense different feeling-tones, some of them slightly painful. Breathe into the pain and let it deepen into nurturing sensations as you exhale. Stroke slowly, sensing fully, with the belly relaxed. Let the breath and the stroke become unified with sensation.

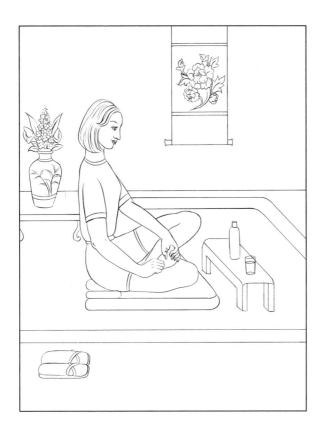

• Arch the toes back with your left hand and jut the heel forward. A valley is formed in the middle of the sole when you do this. Using the knuckles or fist of your right hand, press firmly all the points along this valley. The tendon here may be very tight and sore.

You may feel a sudden surge of energy or a rush of warmth around your heart as you press. Explore sensitively, bringing awareness into whatever feelings that may come up as a result of the masage.

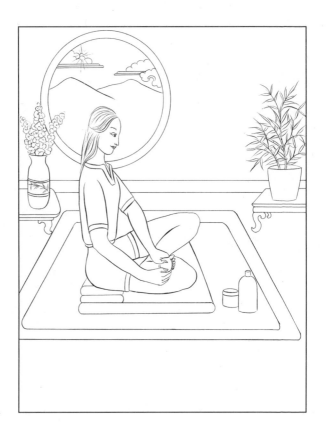

• Grasp one side of the ball of the foot with the left hand and the other side with the right hand. Pull apart as though you were trying to make the sole convex. Maximize the contact of your hands and feet as you pull. Then strongly pull the sides of the feet toward you as if trying to make the sole concave.

• Move to the heel; pinch and probe all areas. Strongly press points 16 and 17 (see Figure 8).

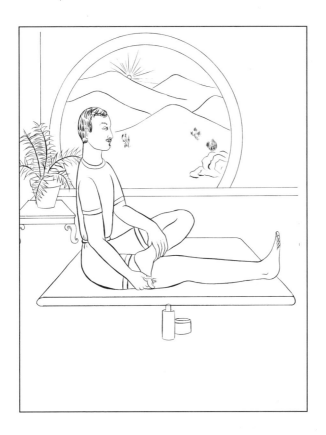

• Grasp the toes of the left foot with your right hand and rest your left hand on the left leg just above the ankle. With your foot relaxed, rotate the ankle in a circle, first in one direction and then in the other. Let your hand do the work; the foot is completely relaxed.

If you feel tight places, explore them by moving more slowly, breathing gently. Let any tensions throughout the body relax. Continue the rotations for several minutes, until they become smooth and easy.

• Pinch and rub vigorously the Achilles' tendon at the back of the foot.

• Apply pressure to all points on and around the ankle. Include ankle points 12 and 13 in Figure 7, (page 135), and points 18–21 in Figure 8 (page 141).

• Position your foot so you can massage the top of it comfortably. Rub between the toes and trace between the tendons, working up to the ankle. Include the sides of the foot in your massage.

• Repeat the foot massage, this time a little more slowly. If there are points at which pressure produces changes in feeling, continue to apply pressure and try to go into the feeling, expanding it as much as possible. If the massage uncovers a sore spot, massage it gently without lingering over it.

Try this simple test. Stand up, resting your weight equally on each foot. How do the two feet relate to the ground? Do you notice any differences? Does one foot feel light, the other heavy? Does there seem to be an energy, an aliveness in one foot in contrast to dullness in the other?

• Now repeat the foot massage on the right foot.

Figure 9 shows an overview of all the pressure points mentioned in this chapter. These pressure points, like all

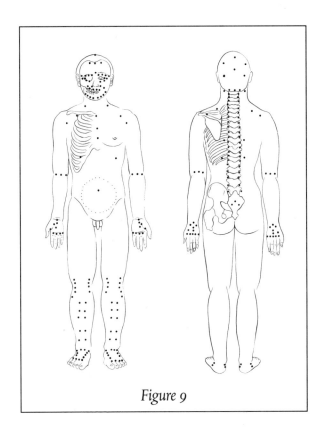

Figure 9

other Kum Nye exercises and massages, are like a map that can guide you in your exploration of the rich inner treasures of your body, mind, and senses. As you become familiar with these points and the special qualities of feeling that pressure on them produces, your understanding of the nature of embodiment will deepen. You may discover additional pressure points in your explorations (even internal ones). As your practice progresses, you may be able to chart your experiences of body and mind, creating maps that will guide others.

147

Guiding Practice

Once you have tasted inner relaxation,
your body will be your truest guide.

Exercises that are genuine and pure, uniting body and mind, truly revitalize our energies and sustain us in our daily lives. We become free from negativity, dissatisfaction, and confusion, for we are able to satisfy ourselves directly instead of chasing after rainbows.

Kum Nye exercises activate a positive healing process that nurtures us mentally and emotionally as well as physically. These exercises are designed to contact the whole body and mind, and in doing so, to unify all its aspects. These are exercises that stimulate body awareness, sensory awareness, and mental awareness, affecting not only the physical systems of the body, but the subtle energy and emotional systems as well. Each exercise loosens physical and psychological tension at the same time, and stimulates feelings that lead to physical and mental balance.

When we give our sensations more flavor, really bringing them into our bodies, we can expand them through our senses and thoughts. When we join breath and awareness to each feeling, it turns into healing, invigorating energy. We may not be able to reach the roots of every feeling at first, but when we make the feelings richer, they grow quickly. If a 'negative' emotion such as resentment or fear arises, we can mix it with our positive sensations and memories, like adding milk to tea. We can make it delicious, give it more flavor, until positive and negative become the same and are equal.

Once the flow of feeling is stimulated, interconnecting all aspects of body and mind, the exercises become opportunities to explore the ease that characterizes the harmonious relationship among body, breath, senses, mind, and environment. The mind and breath support the senses, and the senses in turn support the body, breath, and mind. The body and mind become one.

As our mental and physical energies become vital and sustaining, we grow clear and confident. Our communication becomes more alive. We can live cheerfully and selflessly, with an ever-increasing capacity for enjoyment. We experience the beauty of natural existence and can contact a dimension of experience that we ordinarily are not able to touch.

Our concentration takes on a light, almost floating quality which opens us to broader perspectives of experience. Our inner cosmos becomes a unity which cannot be separated from the outer cosmos. We realize that there are no separate spaces, and all space becomes opent and inviting. As we continue to develop the experience of balance, we develop an open, willing, and accepting attitude toward every aspect of life. All our actions are expressions of a wholesome attitude, and daily life becomes luminous in quality.

This ongoing exercise of body, mind, and senses—this interaction—is called embodiment: a living, continuing process of enjoyment that informs all of our activities. As we feel sensations of inner warmth, thick and rich like fresh cream, a quality of sweetness develops, a deep, gentle quality which continues to increase and refresh itself, fulfilling and nourishing us and those around us. We can expand this quality of enjoyment more and more, until, with time, every movement, every word, and every glance becomes subtle interaction, an exercise.

The ideal way to practice Kum Nye is doing the breathing and movement exercises in the morning and the massage in the evening. Two groups of exercises are included in this section to help you in planning your morning practice during the first few months of practice. Part Two contains many more movement exercises. If you wish to practice only once a day, some massage can easily be added to the movement exercises you choose.

There are ten exercises in each group. The exercises in Group One correspond in difficulty to those in Stage One of Part Two; the exercises in Group Two correspond to those in Stage Two of Part Two. You might spend two or three months of practice on each group. To develop the exercises in Group One, you might first choose two or three exercises out of the ten, and practice each one daily for about fifteen minutes. After a few weeks, you could add one or two more exercises, continuing to practice two or three exercises each day.

After developing the exercises in Group One over a period of two or three months, you might be ready to add exercises from Group Two (one or two at a time) rather than change to a whole new set. Once you have tasted inner relaxation, your body will be your truest guide.

Let your body lead you to the exercises you practice. If you are unused to exercising, be especially gentle and do not try to do too much. Remember: it is the quality of the movement that is most important. If you are pregnant, do the breathing exercises and the gentle movement exercises such as Exercises 18, 22, 24, and 30. If you have had any kind of neck injury, Exercise 17 is not recommended. After a back injury, do not to do the exercises in which the spine bends forward or backward. Use your own judgment; if you practice any of them, move very gently, with awareness. If you have had an operation within the last three or four months, develop the gentler exercises such as those mentioned above.

When you are practicing the exercises, move very slowly and smoothly. This will allow you to be sensitive and alert to variations in feelings and in body processes. Always move with awareness—never mechanically or absent-mindedly—so that you develop the quality of the practice. Breathe evenly through both nose and mouth, so your energies are constantly balanced, and your sensations are stimulated within balance.

Let your senses, feelings, breath, and awareness move in your body and with your body. Rather than directing the eyes outward, try to look inward with the eyes of the senses, into feelings or tension. Gradually sensing will become awareness. Too much seriousness can lead to rigidity, so aim for a quality in your practice that is a combination of lightness and internal awareness.

As you go deeper into your feelings, your experience of relaxation will continue to expand, and your increasing alertness and capacity for enjoyment will give stability to your life. As your body is nourished by your sensations, you become emotionally more healthy, and an uplifting quality develops within your senses.

Group One

Before beginning these exercises (and at various times as you practice them in the next few months), you may find it useful to reread the chapter "Preparation." After doing so, read through the exercises in this group, and when you are drawn to one, try it. You may want to try a number of the exercises, but then go back to two or three you especially like. Develop them for a few weeks before adding more. Remember not to rush. Stay with an exercise until it opens the door to your senses, awakening feelings that heal both your body and mind.

Forty-five minutes is a good length of time to practice, although even twenty minutes will bring results. Begin by spending fifteen to twenty minutes on each exercise. Do an exercise three times and spend two or three minutes or more on each repetition; then sit quietly for five or ten minutes. Later, you may want to practice an exercise for a longer period of time. If you feel strong emotions, sit quietly and relax for a while before exercising. If you do not feel well, be sure not to do too much.

You will find that the exercises in this group release tension in the upper body, especially the shoulders, neck, and head, and in the spine. The stretching exercises such as Exercises 19, 20, and 21 are especially pleasurable in the morning. Do not stretch too much or too quickly; this may strain muscles and cause a heavy, inert state of mind.

Slowly ease into the stretch, breathing evenly through nose and mouth, and develop a quality of lightness. Then feeling and energy are redistributed throughout the body, and you will begin to feel more in your heart.

These simple exercises help us develop the abundant riches of our inner resources in a natural way. Even if nothing in particular appears to be happening while you do an exercise, a change will be gradually occurring in the quality of your daily life. Every aspect of experience will become clearer and more vital. Every activity of the senses—smelling, seeing, hearing, tasting—will become more substantial, full, and alive. Life develops a special, tangy quality.

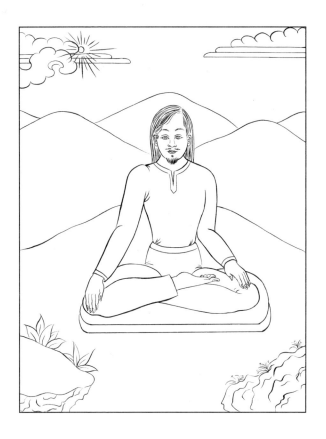

Exercise 15   Loosening Up

Sit cross-legged on a mat or cushion with your hands
on your knees and your arms straight. Facing forward
and breathing easily through both nose and mouth, very
slowly move your shoulders so the right shoulder moves
forward as far as possible and the left shoulder moves
back as far as possible. Keep your right arm straight and
let the left elbow bend. Take about fifteen seconds for
this movement. Then slowly move your left shoulder

forward as your right shoulder moves back, straightening your left arm and allowing your right elbow to bend. Be sure to face forward, so the shoulders move independently of the head. This will feel a little strange at first, for we are accustomed to moving the head and shoulders together. Move very slowly, sensing the feelings awakened in your body. Feel the stretch in your back and neck at the end of the movement; you may feel sensations of warmth there.

Do the complete movement, first one side, then the other, three or nine times. Then sit quietly in the sitting posture for five to ten minutes, distributing the sensations awakened by this movement to your whole body, and beyond, to the universe.

This exercise relaxes the upper back, especially the muscles of the shoulder blades. It also relaxes the hips.

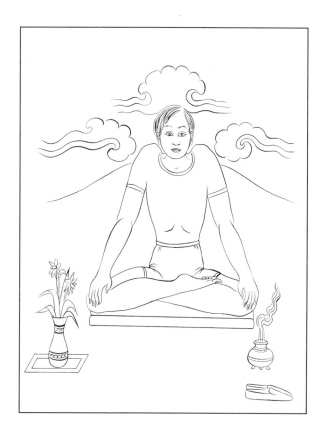

Exercise 16   Touching Feeling

Sit cross-legged on a mat or cushion with your hands on your knees. Relax your belly. Inhale and slowly lift your shoulders as high as possible, allowing the position of your hands to shift as needed.

When you think your shoulders are as high as they can possibly go, relax while still holding them up, and you may find they can be raised a little more. Let your neck settle down between your shoulders.

Now hold your breath a little and lightly imagine the back of your neck, as if it were fresh and warm like that of a happy baby… Then exhale, and in slow motion rotate your shoulders back and down, feeling the sensations in the back of your neck and spine. Keep your belly relaxed. Let your hands and arms be very relaxed—you may feel sensations of warmth and softness there. Slowly continue to rotate your shoulders—forward, up, back, and down— three or nine times. Spend at least one minute on each rotation. Then find a place in the movement where you can comfortably change direction, and make three or nine rotations the other way. At the end, remain in the sitting posture for five to ten minutes, allowing your sensations and feelings to expand.

This exercise can also be done standing. Let your arms hang relaxed and close to your body as you rotate your shoulders in the shoulder joints.

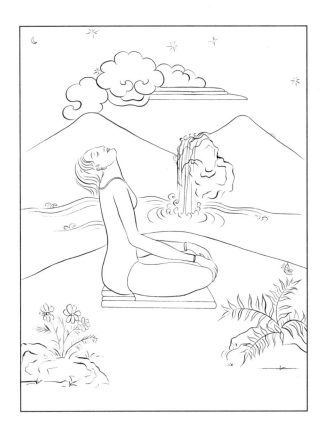

Exercise 17　Lightening Thoughts

If you are pregnant or have had any kind of neck injury, it is best not to do this exercise. Do it especially slowly if your neck muscles are tight. Throughout the exercise breathe very slowly and evenly through both nose and mouth. This is important, for if the breathing is too fast or uneven, this exercise can produce effects such as nausea or disorientation.

Sit cross-legged on a mat or cushion with your hands on your knees. With your mouth opened slightly, breathing gently, very slowly lower your chin toward your chest; then slowly lift the chin until it points toward the ceiling. Repeat this very slow lifting and lowering of the chin several times.

Now very slowly move your head so your right ear moves in the direction of your right shoulder, and then so your left ear moves in the direction of your left shoulder. Repeat several times.

Softly close your eyes and slowly begin to rotate your head clockwise, as if drawing a perfect circle with the top of the head. Relax your shoulders—they should not move with the head. Let the neck muscle open and lengthen, without stretching too much. Make the circle as large and full as you can without straining—let the ears come close to the shoulders, and the chin near the chest. When you feel a tight or painful place, move your head back and forth, allowing the muscles to loosen and lengthen. You may catch a thought related to the tightness. Slow the speed of the rotation down with mind, breath, and senses until the movement is almost imperceptible. Be aware of the whole body, up to the toes and fingertips.

During the rotation, concentrate loosely on the juncture of your skull and spine, under the occiput. You may feel a special energy there, almost a sense of home. Deepen this feeling and expand it as much as you can. Use the spine as a channel for this feeling, distributing it throughout the body. Expand the feeling so it becomes larger than your body and continues to expand outside the body, on and on.

Rotate the head three or nine times in clockwise direction. Find a place in the movement where you feel comfortable changing direction, and begin three or nine counterclockwise rotations. Throughout the movement remember to breathe evenly through nose and mouth.

On the last rotation, move your head more and more slowly until it finally stops moving. Then sit quietly in the sitting posture for ten minutes, continuing to expand your feelings and energy.

This exercise relieves tension in the neck, head, and shoulders and lightens the fixed and usually tight quality of thoughts and images.

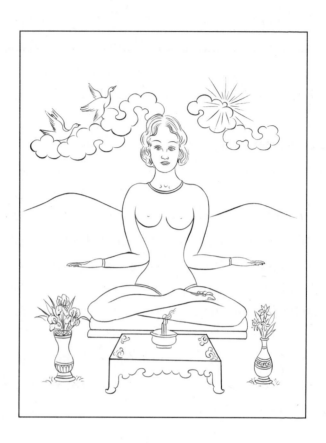

Exercise 18   Hand Magic

This exercise is most effective when done after massaging or after energizing the hands.

Sit cross-legged with your hands on your knees. Slowly lift your arms to chest level, with your elbows bent and your palms down. Relax your elbows and move them away from your body a little. Breathing softly and evenly through both nose and mouth, begin moving your hands up and down a few inches. Move softly, slowly, and casually, until you feel heat underneath the hands, a steady fire. With eyes half-closed, use your peripheral vision to look at the motion. Relax the shoulders and slow down the movement of the hands, until you can hardly see any movement. Can you feel heat in your palms, at the back of the neck, behind the spinal cord, in the chest?

If you do not feel heat, you may be moving too quickly. Let the hands just hang down from your wrists, and relax the elbows. Move lightly, as if touching the texture of space. Make the motion smaller, shorter, softer, gentler. The movement becomes even slower, until it is like a pulsation, almost imperceptible, a tiny bee buzzing. Do the palms feel hot? Do you feel something up and down the fingers? Perhaps a tingling with a special quality?

Once you feel something in your palms or fingers, keep your hands in front of you and slowly turn the palms up, holding them as if they were supporting air. Press the elbows into your sides and push the chest out a little. Keeping the palms up, slowly move your hands toward each other, feeling the sensations of heat and energy; then, before they touch, move them apart and separate them as much as possible. Can you still feel the energy? Your elbows stay in the same position throughout, firmly pressed into your sides. Continue, three or nine times.

With your palms up and your elbows pressed into your sides, now move your hands toward and away from each other in a very fast, short, strong motion. Relax your belly and let strength pass from the shoulders into the hands. Your neck is straight and strong; your hands are shaking as fast as possible. Continue this movement for thirty seconds to one minute.

Gradually slow down the movement of your hands and let them come to rest in your lap, the back of one hand held in the palm of the other, your head bent slightly forward. Relax your shoulders. It is as if your hands encircle the energy and bring it to rest. Sit for five to ten minutes, expanding the sensations in your body. After you have practiced this exercise ten times over a period of a week or two, go on to the following exercises.

• Sit cross-legged with your hands on your knee. Breathe gently and evenly through both nose and mouth. Slowly lift your arms to chest level and begin to move your hands in unison in any way you feel like, sensing energy inside your palms. Try moving them slowly up and down or from side to side. You may feel sensations of coolness or warmth. Feel the energy in different ways. Perhaps lift your hands as if you were raising a heavy lid. Or push something down with great effort. You may be aware of a kind of feeling-form, an energy shape. You may even be able to feel inside the form of the energy.

Now slowly begin to play with the energy. Twist it, pull it, put it together, disperse it, make solid forms—play with it in any way you are moved to do so. As you play, let your

mind become united with the feelings until there is nothing other than these sensations of energy.

Now grip your sides with your elbows, and with your
palms facing each other and the fingers pointing forward,
begin to vibrate your hands rapidly back and forth. (Keep
the fingers of each hand together.) Start with your hands
wide apart and push the energy together, making it dens-
er and stronger. Let strength come from your shoulders
into your hands, so your hands become heavier. Feel the
sensations of energy, the different weights and textures.
You are contacting air as well as energy; behind the air is
the energy. Feel the different qualities of energy—perhaps
a quality like fine cloth, or like drinking water.

Now slowly lessen the movement, and bring your
hands near (without touching) different places on your
body—the top of your head, your throat, your chest, the
area below the navel. Move your hands very slowly and
feel the different qualities of these energy fields. Then
gradually allow your hands to grow still and come to rest
on your knees. Sit quietly for several minutes, feeling the
energies of this 'hand magic'.

Over a period of several weeks, do this exercise twenty-five times, for ten minutes each session. Then you will
become familiar with these different qualities of energy.

• When you have have become familiar with one of the
preceding exercises and feel energy in the hands, rub the

palms together vigorously and distribute the heat energy generated by this motion to the rest of your body, even to each organ. Rub very quickly and strongly with light concentration. Draw your hands up close to your chin and look directly at them as you rub, breathing gently through both nose and mouth. Rub faster and faster, passing the energy into your body.

Now slow the movement down and make it heavier. Slowly cover your eyes with your palms without actually touching the eyes. Feel the energy pass into your eyes. Sit quietly for three to five minutes with your hands over your eyes, feeling the movement of energies within. You may feel sensations in many parts of your body. Let your breath merge with the sensations and amplify them.

When you release your hands, very slowly open your eyes, and look around in a gentle, open way. Do you notice something different, perhaps a feeling or quality? What is the quality of your breathing?

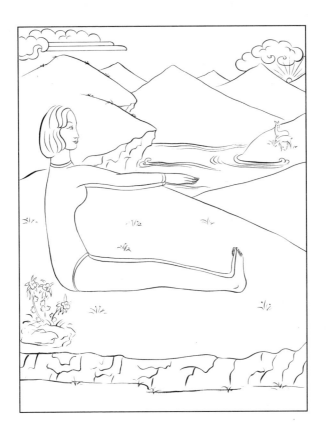

Exercise 19   Revitalizing Energy

Sit on the floor, not on a mat or cushion, with your legs
stretched out in front of you and a comfortable distance
apart, your back straight, and your hands on your knees.
Flex your ankles so your toes point toward your face, and
keep them in this position throughout the movement.
Slowly lift your arms in front of you to shoulder height,
with the palms down. Reach forward toward your toes,
lowering the head between the arms. When you have

167

reached as far as you can without straining (it does not matter how far you reach), very slowly draw back, keeping your arms stretched out in front of you, allowing the head to come up until you are leaning slightly backwards.

Then again reach forward, unhurriedly, toward your toes, without straining. Move even more slowly as you draw back, expanding the sensations that arise. Feel the qualities of space and time. Remember to breathe gently and evenly through both nose and mouth throughout the entire movement.

Repeat the exercise three or nine times. Then remain in the sitting posture for five to ten minutes, breathing gently, amplifying the sensations until they fill the space around you.

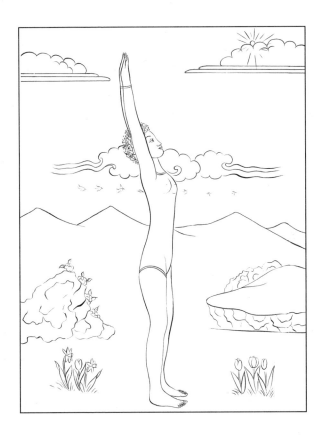

Exercise 20   Touching Body Energy

This exercise is not recommended if you are pregnant or have had any back or neck injuries.

Stand with your feet a comfortable distance apart, your back straight, and your body balanced. Breathing softly through both nose and mouth, slowly raise your arms in front of you until they are overhead, with palms facing forward. With your knees relaxed and straight but not locked, slowly bend forward from the waist while reaching out slightly with your arms. This bending has a quality of arching. Bend forward and down, very slowly and evenly; head, torso, and arms move together. Release tension in your chest, belly, and lower energy centers as you go down.

Do not let your head dominate the movement; relax your neck muscles so your head hangs freely and loosely. Feel the sensations in the back of your body, especially your spine and the backs of your legs. Your knees are straight. When your fingers approach the floor, stay down for a moment, concentrating lightly on your back. Be very still. Spread your fingers apart more. Exhale fully, releasing tension from the belly so the flow of energy is not blocked.

Now very slowly, breathing evenly and gently, begin to rise, keeping your head between your arms. Bring your attention to your throat as you come up—you may feel a sensation of opening there. When you are in upright position, continue to bend slightly backward, with your arms quite close to the head. Move very gently, with your knees straight and your belly and lower organs relaxed. Bend backward only a little, without straining. In this position, keep your exhalations gentle and let the front of your body feel open, especially your belly, chest, and throat.

Slowly straighten your neck and back, bringing your attention to the base of your skull; perhaps you will feel warmth there or a sense of connection and peace as if you had finally come home.

Again bend forward as before, moving as gently and slowly as possible, relaxing your belly, neck, and back. Develop the healing quality of the forward movement, focusing especially on the lower part of your spine. Feel the opening and freeing of the vertebrae. During the first part of the bend, you may be most aware of your upper back. As you bend further, you may feel the middle part of the back opening. As you hands are approaching the floor and the bend is greatest, healing energy may be strongest in your lower back.

When you begin to rise the movement is almost imperceptible, and you can sense the subtle tensions you are holding in your body. When you locate a tension, explore it with your feelings as completely as you can. Perhaps you will find an attitude or an aspect of your self-image within the tightness. When you fully experience the tightness, you will be able to let it go.

As you move, become one with your feelings; let them move you, spreading their energy to every molecule in the body. Finally, you may have the sense that 'you' no longer exist. Instead, there is only feeling.

Repeat the exercise three or nine times. Then remain quietly in the sitting posture for five to ten minutes, expanding the sensations awakened by this movement.

This exercise relieves tension in the back of the neck, the spine, and the backs of the legs, and redistributes energy and feeling throughout the body.

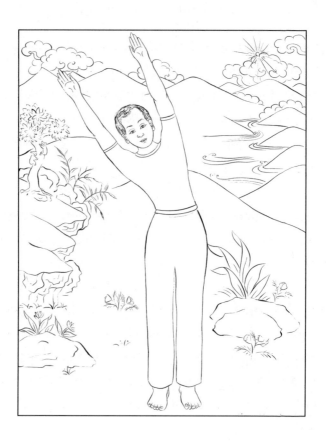

Exercise 21 Healing Body and Mind

Stand with your body well balanced, your feet about a foot apart, your back straight, and your arms relaxed at your sides. Inhale through both nose and mouth and lift your arms in front of you until they are overhead, with the palms facing forward. While exhaling, slowly bend to the right side, reaching out with your arms and keeping your knees straight but not locked. As you bend, let your pelvis move slightly to the left, so your weight is balanced on both feet and the curve on both sides of your body is as long and graceful as possible. Loosen the muscles of the waist, neck, and shoulders, and allow your left hip and the ribs on the left side to open like a fan. Let your left arm come close to your ear, and let your right arm lower a little toward the ground. Keep your mouth slightly open, and let your breath flow evenly.

While inhaling, slowly return to an upright position and in a continuous motion reach to the opposite side while exhaling. Let your belly be relaxed and empty. Move as gradually as you can, feeling the sensations within your body. Do the complete movement, to the right and left, three or nine times, relaxing more each time. Then sit in the sitting posture for five to ten minutes, expanding the feelings stimulated by the exercise. This movement can also be done with the palms facing each other.

This exercise relieves tension in the muscles along the sides of the body.

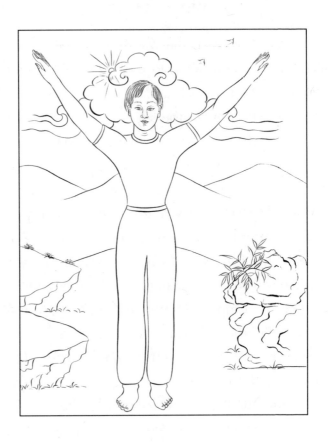

Exercise 22   Flying

Stand well balanced with your feet about four inches apart, the back straight, and the arms relaxed at your sides. Lift your arms away from your sides until they are directly overhead with the backs of the hands almost touching and the fingers straight. Close your eyes and feel the sensations of energy in your body. Relax your thighs and minimize any backward arching in the spine. Open your arms, increasing the distance between them in a balanced and equal way, and gradually let them descend to your sides. Take one full minute to bring them all the way down. Pay attention to the feeling tone as you move, as if seeing with the inner eyes of the senses. Let energy flow into your heart center. As the arms descend to your sides, you may feel heat and energy surrounding your arms and hands.

Now take another full minute to move your arms up again. Explore the flow of energy: you might try directing energy from your heart center out through your fingers. Use the steady, slow rhythm to increase the energy flow. When the arms are overhead, stretch up slightly, with your thighs and legs fully relaxed. This stretch clears and settles the mind; go deeply into your sensations at this point.

Continue the movement nine times. Try slowing the movement down even more, taking at least two minutes in each direction. To complete the exercise, sit in the seven gesture for five minutes or more, continuing to sense the flow of energy, with breath, body, and mind as one.

This exercise calms the restless flow of thoughts and generates feelings in the heart center.

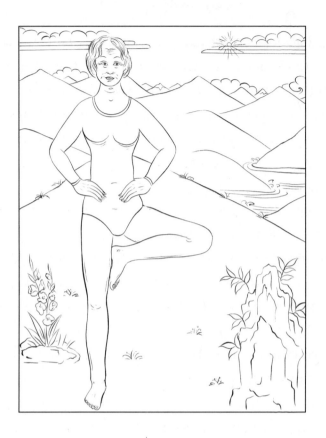

Exercise 23 Balancing Body and Mind

Stand barefoot on the floor with your feet a comfortable distance apart and your back straight. Without hurrying, lift your left leg, bending it at the knee. Grasp the inside of the leg near the ankle with your left hand, and place the sole of your left foot, toes down, against the inside of your upper right thigh, with the heel near the crotch. Press the heel lightly into the thigh to hold your leg in position. Move the left knee out to the side, place your hands on the hips, look straight ahead with soft eyes, and balance casually in this position, concentrating lightly. Distribute some of your weight to your left knee, and loosen your belly. Remain in this position for one to three minutes. Without changing position or losing your balance, slowly reduce the pressure of your left foot against your right thigh until it is almost imperceptible.

Now slowly lift your foot from your thigh and lower your leg to the floor, paying special attention to the sensations you feel just before your left foot touches the ground. Slowly resume a standing position balanced on both legs, then repeat the movement on the other side of your body. Notice on which side balance is easier.

Do the complete movement, both sides, three times. Then sit for ten to fifteen minutes, allowing the sensations stimulated by the posture to expand. Try to follow the process of coming back to a more familiar state of mind. Do you come back in a balanced way?

If you regularly practice this exercise (or any exercise in Part Two in which you balance on one leg), you will find that different feeling states produce different feeling-tones within balance. You will probably find it more difficult to balance when you are emotional, and tightness in your body may make you lose your balance. Relax into the exercise and go deeply into the feelings awakened within you.

This exercise stretches the upper leg and stimulates energy in the sacrum and spine.

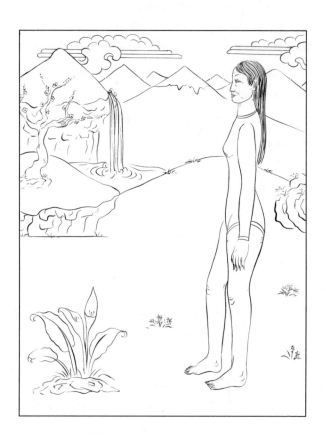

Exercise 24   Being and Body

Stand well balanced with your feet a comfortable distance apart, the back straight, and the arms relaxed at your sides. Breathe softly through nose and mouth. Close your eyes and let tension ebb from your entire body, especially the chest and throat. Take time to sense how tiny adjustments in muscles and energy may affect your balance.

Now slowly open your eyes, look straight ahead, and begin to walk unhurriedly, with very small steps, as few as two inches and not more than four. Walk as slowly as you can imagine walking. Then slow down even more.

Each movement of walking can be an opportunity for learning. Before lifting a foot, relax the belly and chest. At the moment of stepping, relax the knees, belly, and chest. Relax also the fingers and toes, skin, even the bones—let every part of your body be calm and warm. Step lightly and create balance at every moment . . . Balance both sides of your body, balance your concentration, balance your breath. You may then discover that your body moves gracefully and gently by itself.

Between lifting and stepping there is a kind of silence. Tension in the energy centers, especially in the throat center, may block this silent quality. So at the moment of lifting the foot off the ground, relax your throat, as well as your belly, knees, shoulders, hands, and spine. Relax also your way of being aware, so your concentration is not too strong or focused. Then at the crucial point between lifting and stepping, you are balanced, relaxed, and silent.

Give the same emphasis and the same amount of time to each part of the movement—lifting, moving, stepping. Open your senses in such a way that you do not focus on any particular sense. You are no more aware of seeing than of hearing. Give as much power to your feelings as to your eyes, ears, and thoughts.

Feel as much as you think. Give all aspects of the experience equal weight, letting your body and senses operate as a complete whole. As you walk in this way, be aware of the mantra OM AH HUM. You do not need to actually pronounce it; listen to it inwardly.

Practice this slow pace for forty-five minutes, moving so slowly that you cover ten yards, back and forth, four times. The next time you practice, walk half as slowly, covering ten yards, back and forth, two times in forty-five minutes.

• Once you have practiced this slow, balanced, walking for three hours, try some variations. Imagine you are working somewhere, perhaps at your office. You want to get home and you are a little late. Close your eyes and feel that urge: "I have to get home quickly." Now walk with that feeling. How do you move? How does your body feel? Now slow down, and walk very slowly for one minute. Notice any differences in your inner body senses.

Now try another way. Imagine you must catch a plane for an important family engagement. You have to get there quickly. Your mind is extremely busy and rushed, and you wish to go faster, but your body moves very, very slowly. Walk, trying to feel equally the anxiety and the slowing down, the very fast and the very slow.

Now intensify the anxiety so you are almost shaking. You want to catch that plane, but you cannot get there. Your mind is agitated because you cannot have what you want. Develop great mental anxiety, a mixture of intense frustration and pain, almost anger. Slow your pace down even more. Which parts of your body are most tense? Are your hands, chest, and stomach loose? Relax tense places without releasing the strong mental pressure. Can you keep your breathing at an even level?

Now try walking very fast. Your body is rushed and yet your mind, awareness, and breath are calm, moving at very slow speed. Breath and awareness are almost silent. You are not trying either to breathe or to be aware.

Now slow down and walk quietly. Can you equalize the speeds of the body, the breathing, and awareness? Can your body, breath, and awareness be equally silent and slow, without special emphasis? What is the quality of the energy you feel?

Group Two

At this point in your practice, you have already begun to touch and develop sensations that relax, nurture, and satisfy you. The exercises in this group will help you to deepen these experiences, and will also introduce new feeling-tones which can be extended and enriched.

As you practice, continue to pay attention to the flavors of feeling each exercise stimulates. Let the body guide you in combining exercises and in developing sequences of exercises. Do not try to name or label the feeling-tones of your experience; simply feel. Become acquainted with the qualities: their texture and weight, their sense of time. You may not have the vocabulary to describe the subtle feeling-tones, but you can experience them.

After spending a few weeks on these exercises, you may feel ready to look at some of the exercises in Part Two (starting on page 208). The exercises in Stages One and Two of Part Two will continue to extend the process of relaxation you have already begun; the exercises in Stage Three will give you an idea of how Kum Nye yoga can be further developed. Be sure, however, not to move too quickly into Part Two, or to practice too many exercises at once. Add one or two exercises to those in this group, and develop them fully before going on to more. Then your practice will have a clear, stable quality, and you will develop trust in your experience.

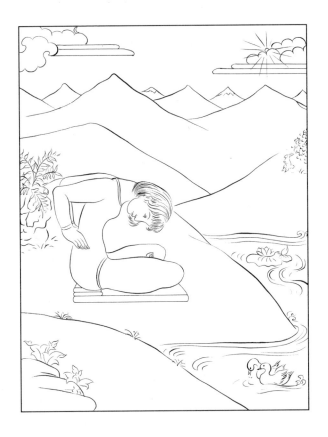

Exercise 25   Calming Inner Energy

Sit cross-legged on a cushion with your back straight
and the hands on your hips. Move your upper body in a
circle, bending slowly to your left from the waist. Breathe
through both nose and mouth, the head and neck relaxed
and hanging. Then, unhurriedly, move forward so your
head skims your left knee, passes close to the ground and
then skims your right knee. Move up on the right side,
then arch backward slightly, looking toward the ceiling.

Without stopping, continue the circle to the left, moving slowly and maintaining balance. Your mouth should be relaxed and slightly open. Fully exhale in the lower position and breathe normally and gently during the rest of the rotation.

After nine clockwise rotations, slowly change directions and continue for nine counterclockwise rotations. This exercise may bring you to a still place where you have few or no thoughts. If this happens, slow the movement down even more, expanding this feeling. When you finish the exercise, sit in the sitting posture for five to ten minutes, continuing to follow and extend the sensations stimulated by the movement.

• This exercise may also be done standing. Stand well balanced with your hands on your hips, your feet about a foot apart, your knees straight but not locked, and your back straight. Feel a column of energy within your body. Bend forward from your waist, to waist level or somewhat lower, letting your head hang, and very slowly begin to rotate your upper body in a clockwise circle around the inner column of energy. The revolution should be complete and continuous, although you arch backward much less than you bend forward. Do not strain; relax and let gravity lead you down. Let your belly, neck, shoulders, and jaw be relaxed. Breathe easily through both nose and mouth. Very slowly, make three or nine clockwise circles, then three or nine counterclockwise circles. Bring a light concentration to the sensations traveling down your spine as you move; feel them more. Let your concentration encompass the pelvis as well—light concentration here will help to support the body and increase the flow of energy. Feel the balancing of the inner column. When you finish the rotations, sit in the sitting posture for five to ten minutes, exploring the sensations stimulated by this movement.

• Another version of this exercise: stand well balanced with feet about a foot apart and your arms relaxed at your sides. Slowly lift your arms away from your sides until they are overhead and turn the palms to face each other. Imagine that your hands are carrying a large ball of energy. In this position, continuing to imagine the ball carried in your hands, bend forward at the waist to about waist level, and begin to rotate your upper body in a clockwise circle. Concentrate lightly on your pelvis and the sensations moving down your spine.

Feel energy flowing from the ball of energy through your hands, arms, and head, passing down your spine. Become the ball of energy, moving through space. Make three or nine clockwise circles, then three or nine counterclockwise circles, all very slow. To complete the exercise, sit in the sitting posture for five to ten minutes, expanding the feelings within and around the body. These exercises calm the internal organs and the nervous system.

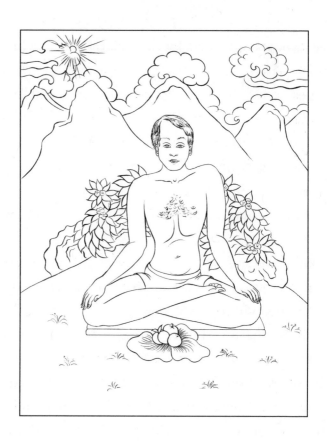

Exercise 26   Stimulating Inner Energy

Sit cross-legged on a mat or cushion with your back straight and your hands on your knees. Bring your attention to your navel area, and slowly begin to move your belly in a circle, up on the right and down on the left. Do the movement attentively, entering into the sensations stimulated by it. Notice that as your belly makes a circle, your chest also moves in a circle. Breathe softly through both nose and mouth, and let the slow circling movement of your belly and chest become ever fuller and deeper, so the movement gives a massage to the internal organs as well as the sides of your body. Continue for several minutes, until the feeling of the massage becomes almost tangible. Try a few circles in the other direction.

Now slow the movement down even more, until the massage is stimulated more by feeling-tone than by actual movement. Let body, breath, and mind become one. Gradually the movement lessen until you finally stop moving. Sit quietly and let the massage of feeling permeate every part of your body and continue for as long as possible. The longer the feeling-tone is expanded, the more the massage moves beyond the body, stimulating interactions with the surrounding universe.

When the feeling-tone begins to fade, experiment with ways to stimulate the belly and chest massage without actually moving physically. Try turning the belly around like a ball with the breath. Also try moving the belly up and down with the breath. You can also experiment with activating the massage through concentration only, as if the senses were rubbing themselves internally.

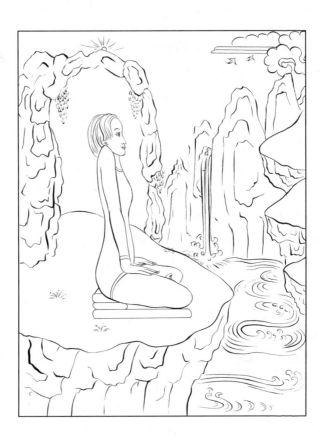

Exercise 27   Touching Nurturing Feeling

Sit comfortably on a mat or cushion in a cross-legged position, with the knees wide apart and the back straight. Place your hands on the top of your upper thighs, with the fingers pointing forward. In this position, slowly push your hands against your thighs so your arms straighten and both shoulders are lifted as high as possible. When you think your shoulders are as high as they can be, relax your body, and you may find your shoulders can move up a little more. Settle your neck down between the shoulders; the chin will almost touch your chest. Breathe lightly through nose and mouth, with your throat and belly as relaxed as possible. Hold this posture for three to five minutes (you can measure time with the out-breath), raising energy from the belly into the chest. Keep the energy high, 'holding' it in a balanced way.

After three to five minutes, very slowly loosen your shoulders a little. Do not rotate the shoulders as they loosen; simply release the tension little by little and allow the shoulders to move down in the same vertical plane. The elbows will begin to bend as the arms relax. Take at least one minute for the release. Feel energy flowing down the length of your spine, from the neck to the lower back and sacrum. When you first do this exercise, the energy will flow down the spine, then forward and up inside your body to the throat, then back and down the spine. Later you will be able to move the energy in every direction, to all parts of your body.

Now modify the exercise lightly. Push your hands against your thighs, straighten your elbows, and lift your shoulders as before, but this time make your belly a little smaller, and tighten the back of the spine slightly. It may seem that you are trying to control the breath, but instead just breathe slowly through both nose and mouth. Remain still and hold the posture for three to five minutes. If you feel a little pain in the neck, upper shoulders, or lower back, carefully move your shoulders slightly so energy can flow smoothly there.

After three to five minutes, very slowly relax the tension and feel the deep, sensitive feeling that arises. Let the tension go completely from your arms in a natural way— very gradually and slowly. Take your time. You may feel warmth in your chest and the back of your neck or a sensation of opening in your chest, throat, and head, a feeling of expanding beyond your body. Do the exercise three or nine times. Be as relaxed and open as possible, not holding back, not specifically focused on achieving anything.

To complete the exercise, sit for ten to fifteen minutes, expanding the sensations generated by holding and releasing tension.

This exercise stretches all the muscles and ligaments between the bones of the upper body, especially the upper part of the spine, and circulates energy to the spine and joints. It can also be done standing.

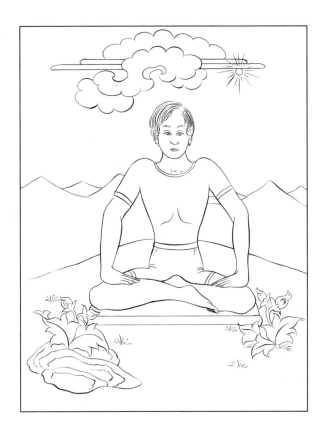

Exercise 28   Body of Knowledge

If you have had a back or neck injury or have had an operation within three or four months, move carefully in this
exercise and do less than the directions indicate.

Sit cross-legged on a mat or cushion, with the pelvis higher than the legs. Place your hands on your knees
so the fingers point towards each other, with the fingers
and thumb of each hand together. The elbows point out
to the side. Slowly arch your head forward and down so

191

the chin moves toward the chest. Unhurriedly bend forward from the waist, pressing the hands firmly against the knees, and pushing the elbows forward a little. Gently pull the belly back against the spine and hold it tightly, breathing softly and evenly through nose and mouth.

Each time you exhale, let each section of the spine—between your shoulder blades, the middle back, the lower back, at the sacrum—open and expand. You may feel as if space opens between each vertebra, and even within each spinal bone. When you have bent forward as far as you can without straining, focus lightly on the base of your spine; you may feel an opening there, as well as a sensation of warmth.

Expand these feelings as much as you can, up your spine and throughout your body. Remain down for three to five minutes. (You can measure the time by counting out-breaths.)

Just before you begin to come up, change the hand position so the fingers and thumbs point straight ahead. Come up and press the hands strongly against the legs. The tension may cause mild shaking; stay with the shaking and notice feelings. You may move beyond shaking to a plateau where the shaking continues but the breath becomes tranquil and soft. At that point the mind has a crystal quality. Slowly release the tension and sit still for five minutes, expanding the feelings. Repeat the movement three or nine times, sitting for five minutes after each repetition. To complete the exercise, sit for ten to fifteen minutes, continuing to expand the sensations within and around your body.

To develop this exercise further, stay down for longer periods of time, up to twenty minutes (in such a case, do it only once), and sit afterward for the same length of time you stayed down.

This exercise relieves eyestrain and general tiredness. It also helps to build muscles and to improve the functioning of the joints.

• This variation of the above exercise is a little more difficult. Sit on a mat or cushion with your legs loosely crossed. The position of your legs will affect your balance in doing this exercise, so you may want to experiment with different ways of crossing them until you find the position that permits the most balanced movement.

Interlace your fingers and place them on the back of your neck, keeping your elbows out. Slowly push your neck down with your hands so your chin moves toward your chest. In this position, bend forward from the waist, breathing lightly and evenly through both nose and mouth, with your belly held tightly against your spine. As you exhale, let each part of the spine open and expand. When you have bent forward as far as you can without straining, focus lightly on the base of your spine, allowing the sensations there to spread out like a halo.

Then, without holding the position, come up as slowly as you can. As the spine straightens, hold some strength in the muscles of your chest, as if directing an energy flow through your chest up into your throat. Then slowly lower your hands to your knees and sit for a few minutes, breathing gently and evenly through both nose and mouth.

Do this exercise three or nine times, sitting for a few moments after each repetition. At the end, sit for five to ten minutes, continuing to expand the sensations at the base of your spine and in your chest and throat, until they are distributed throughout the body and become part of the space that surrounds you. Let the feelings spread out like a mandala.

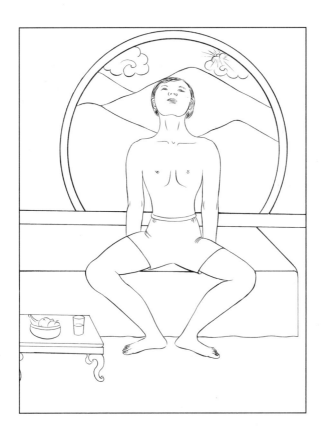

Exercise 29   Clear Light

Do this exercise gently if you are pregnant, if you have had any sort of back or neck injury, or an operation within three or four months.

Sit on the edge of a straight chair with your feet flat on the floor about six inches apart, the heels pointing toward each other and the toes pointing out. Place your hands in back of you on the chair with the fingers pointing behind you. Breathing lightly through both nose and mouth, press your hands down and arch your spine and neck backward, letting the mouth fall open. Hold for thirty seconds to three minutes; then very, very slowly straighten the neck and back, sensing the feelings stimulated by the posture. You may feel heat in the back of your neck and the base of your spine.

Sit with your hands on your knees for a few minutes, distributing these sensations throughout your body. Then repeat the exercise two more times, sitting for five to ten minutes at the end.

A variation of this exercise is done with the hands next to the hips on the side of the chair, with the fingers pointing forward.

This exercise can relieve ulcers and stomach pain, as well as psychological tensions.

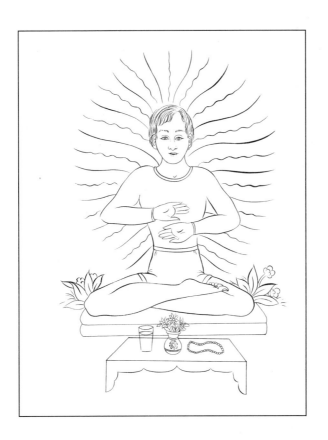

Exercise 30   Expanding Awareness

Sit cross-legged on a mat or cushion and place your hands in your lap with the palms up, the right hand held in the left. Loosen your belly and chest, settle your neck down between your shoulders, and relax tension in your spine. Gracefully lift your arms overhead, finishing with the palms facing forward. Imagine a huge ball of energy in front of you. Slowly open your arms and move them down in lateral arcs as if encircling this ball of energy with your hands. Feel the sensations of energy in your hands and arms that this movement stimulates.

As you round the bottom of the ball, with palms up, cross the right wrist over the left without touching them together. In a continuing movement, twist both wrists until the palms face away from you. Keeping the hands in the same plane, draw them toward each other slightly. Without ceasing the movement, slowly and gracefully lift the arms in front of you. First the right arm, and as soon as there is enough room, the left arm, keeping elbows and hands relaxed. Move your arms up until they are both outstretched overhead, and the movement, with its special design, has begun again.

Repeat the movement three or nine continuous times. With each repetition relax more deeply, allowing the sensations awakened to spread throughout your body. Breathe very softly through both nose and mouth, with your belly and chest relaxed. Then adapt the 'rounding the ball' movement to bring your hands to rest on your knees. Sit for five to ten minutes, continuing to expand the sensations of energy within and outside of your body.

This exercise expands awareness and concentration and releases tension in the upper back and shoulders. Try it after sitting for fifteen to thirty minutes.

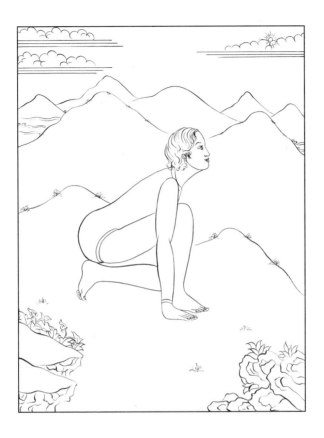

Exercise 31   Knowing Only Bliss

Kneel on the ground with your thighs vertical. Lift your right knee and place your right foot on the floor, with the toes a few inches to the right of your left knee. Sit back on your left heel and bring your right heel to the floor. (You will keep your right foot flat on the floor throughout the movement). Place the palms flat on the floor, the left palm a few inches to the left of the left knee, and the right palm a few inches to the right of the right foot, so the hands, knee and foot are in a line. Now lower your head and lift your pelvis so you can stand on the toes of your left foot. Be alert and sensitive to these toes during the exercise, so you do not put too much weight on them.

In this position, keeping your palms flat on the floor, lift your chest as much as possible, and look up toward the ceiling. Hold for fifteen to thirty seconds, breathing gently through both nose and mouth and concentrating lightly on your back. Then lower the head and let it hang loosely. Now lift the pelvis slightly and strongly press with both hands, your left knee and your right foot to the ground. Hold for fifteen to thirty seconds, breathing easily through both nose and mouth. Slowly release the tension, straighten your left foot, and sit in the sitting posture for a few minutes.

Now reverse the position of the legs and repeat the exercise. Do the complete movement, first on one side, then on the other, three times, resting briefly after each repetition. Finally, sit quietly for five to ten minutes, expanding the sensations stimulated within and around you.

This exercise relieves tension in the neck and stimulates energy in the lower back that then flows up the back and through the neck.

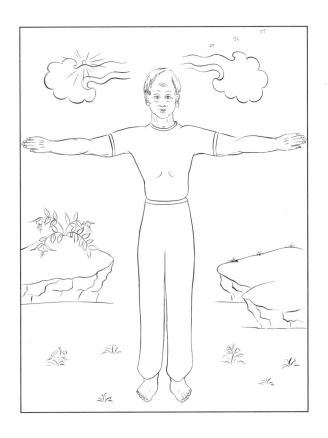

Exercise 32   Touching Body, Mind, and Energy

Stand well balanced with your feet a comfortable distance apart, your back straight, and your arms relaxed at your sides. Slowly raise your arms in front of you to a little above shoulder height, with your hands about two inches apart, the backs of the hands facing each other and the fingers straight. Picture steel bars next to your palms and begin to move your arms out to the sides, as if you were pushing these steel bars apart. Push with strength until the outstretched arms are a little behind your shoulders. Breathe lightly and evenly through nose and mouth. Keep your belly, chest, and thighs relaxed and concentrate lightly on the base of the spine. If the muscles of the upper and middle back are painful and tense, move more gently.

Now imagine that the steel bars are near the backs of your hands, and slowly move your hands toward the front, as if you were pushing the bars together. Notice the different quality of the movement in this direction. Feel the energy surrounding your hands and arms, while still concentrating loosely on the base of the spine.

Release the tension in your arms very slowly, lowering them to your sides. Stand for two minutes, expanding the sensations of energy. Then continue the exercise, three or nine times, standing with your arms at your sides after each repetition. When you finish, sit for five minutes or more, sensing the energy flow in your body.

This exercise increases circulation and awareness, and will invigorate you when you feel tired, sleepy, or clumsy.

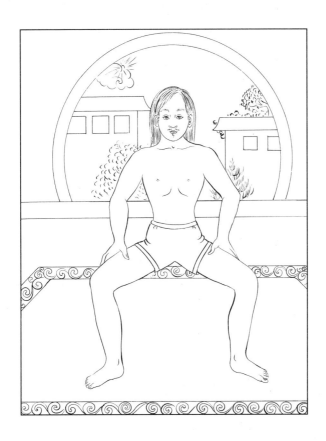

Exercise 33　Energizing the Lower Body

Stand well balanced with your back straight, your legs
wide apart, and your toes turned out slightly. Place your
hands on your thighs, with your thumbs toward the inside
of the leg. Breathe softly through both nose and mouth;
relax your shoulders, and look straight ahead with the
back straight. In this position, bend your knees and lower
your pelvis until you find a place where energy is strongly
activated in the legs (they may shake). Move up and down

a little or move your legs closer or wider apart to find it. Keep your weight evenly distributed on both feet and your back straight.

As you move down, you may find that tension somewhere prevents you from moving further. Locate this tension, gently release it, and continue to lower. Use the exercise to explore subtle tensions which interfere with balance and the even flow of energy in your body.

Once you find the right place, remain in this position for fifteen seconds, with the genital and anal areas open and relaxed, and breathing softly. You will feel pressure on the knees. After fifteen seconds, slowly straighten your legs, move your feet closer together, relax your arms at your sides, and stand or sit for a few minutes, expanding the feelings quickened by the exercise.

Do the exercise three times, resting after each repetition; then sit in the sitting posture for five to ten minutes, continuing to amplify and extend the sensations in your body. As you become more familiar with this exercise, try holding the position for longer periods of time. Also experiment with inhaling as you move down and exhaling as you come up.

This exercise tends to release energy blockages in the lower body.

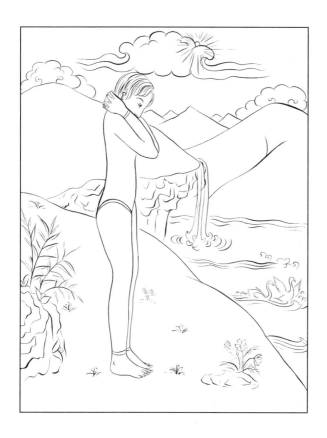

Exercise 34   Inner Gold

Stand well balanced with your feet about six inches apart and your back straight. Interlace your fingers and place them at the back of your neck, so they support your head. Slowly push your neck back against your hands, spread your elbows apart as wide as possible, bend your knees slightly, and lift your chest toward the ceiling. The lower part of your spine should be as relaxed as possible, while your upper spine arches backwards. Remaining in this position, exhale slowly and deeply for as long as you can. Feel the stretch in the muscles under your arms and at the sides of your chest. Go deeply into the sensations that arise in your chest.

Now, while inhaling, slowly and steadily press your hands against the back of your neck, bending your neck forward and lowering your elbows until the chin is near the chest and the elbows hang down close together. As you reach this lowered position, hold the breath a little and relax the muscles of your shoulders and upper back. Then continuing to inhale, slowly push your neck against your hands, move your elbows wide apart, and lift your chest toward the ceiling, allowing it to open. Exhale in the open position.

Continue this opening and folding movement three or nine times, as slowly as can be coordinated with your breathing. Then sit in the sitting posture for ten minutes, expanding the sensations stimulated by the exercise.

As you experience more openness physically in the heart area, you may feel a deep, open, loving feeling arise that can be distributed to all parts of your body and can expand beyond your body to the surrounding universe. This exercise can also relieve pain and tension in the stomach area.

Part Two

MOVEMENT EXERCISES

Balancing and Integrating Body, Mind, and Senses

Balance is a natural condition of flowing feeling
and energy that pervades the entire body and mind.

We commonly think of balance as our bodily equilibrium or stability. This understanding of balance is limited, however, and can be expanded by certain exercises and movements which show us how bring our breath, senses, and awareness into balance with our bodies and minds. We can make our whole system balanced, for balance is a natural condition of flowing feeling and energy which pervades entire body and mind. This balance is the objective of Kum Nye.

The foundation of balance and the integration of body and mind is relaxation. Often we think of relaxation as a state of dreaminess, lacking in awareness and vitality; or a process of escaping from life; or a filling or a marking out of time. But true relaxation is actually balance. When we are relaxed, we open to new sensory fields and dimensions, expanding sensations and feelings that bring body and mind together. We learn to generate and accumulate energy, using it so both body and mind work together in a flowing, open way. Thoughts and sensations flow more smoothly as the mind is vibrant and clear and the body vital and energetic. When we truly relax, it is no longer the 'self' that is experiencing—we become the experience itself. We no longer 'own' our senses, bodies, and minds, for they all totally participate in the experience.

Often, however, our minds and bodies do not communicate well with each other. In a similar case we are unable to nourish either one properly. We cannot sustain our vitality, concentration, or awareness, so we function ineffectively and become prone to mental as well as physical imbalances. Most psychological problems and most illnesses—including the diseases of stress—are related to the subtle energy imbalances in our bodies, minds, and senses. Our sensations become confused and our energy scattered and unsteady. Lacking vital awareness, the body and senses are like unused houses: mental, physical, and sensory awareness diminish. Strong emotions aggravate the situation.

The integration and balancing of physical and mental energies free us from such patterns. We become able to flow with experience, allowing it to nourish and satisfy us. Our perspective changes, and we learn to understand things in new ways—we see that neither the good nor the bad experiences last for long, and we become less subject to emotional extremes. We do not try to control or fix our experience, for we possess a knowledge based on opening to each situation in our lives as an opportunity for growth. We open to the vital and wholesome nature of all experience, and see the preciousness and grace of every aspect of life. Our peacefulness shows us the harmony of existence, and everything becomes relevant to our lives. We come to appreciate every person, situation, sensation, and feeling in our lives, even those we call 'negative'.

When our relationships to the world become more and complete, our ability to communicate improves, and we are less dependent on others to protect our sense of well-being and happiness. We become willing to expand beyond the limited space and time of our usual sense of 'privacy', expanding our senses, feelings, thoughts, and awareness. Eventually we discover an infinite sort of knowledge that itself can be extended and that gives us a way of understanding the beauty, richness, and value of our inner resources.

The exercises in this chapter are divided into three stages. There is a progression within each stage, and from stage to stage. If you wish, do the exercises in the order they are presented; however, do not feel that you must do them in this progression. Some exercises will suit you better than others, and it is perfectly all right to do the exercises within a stage in a different sequence, or to practice some of the exercises in Stage Two or even Stage Three before doing all of the exercises in Stage One. Feel free to experiment with different combinations of exercises. Let your body lead you to those exercises that stimulate the most vital feeling for you, and vary the sequence and combination of exercises enough so that your practice is interesting and balanced.

If you can, allow forty-five minutes a day for practice; if you cannot spare that much time, twenty to thirty minutes will also bring results. Begin by practicing two or three exercises each day, doing each exercise three times. Choose three or four exercises that you like, and stay with them until you feel confident you have touched your feelings deeply. This may take two or three weeks. Then over the next six or eight weeks, gradually increase your vocabulary of exercises to approximately ten. Practice some of the standing exercises as well as the sitting ones; at times you may want to do some massage or a breathing exercise along with the movement exercises.

Whatever sequence or combination of exercises you choose, do not be in a rush. Coverage and speed are not important. Remember that these exercises are different from ordinary physical exercises; they are not designed simply to improve the physical functioning of the body. They will do this, but when practiced properly, they will also awaken the senses, stimulating certain feeling-tones which, when cultivated and extended, improve the functioning of the total organism—body, mind, and senses.

Each exercise is a symbol that leads to special energies or feeling tones. As you practice an exercise, develop the qualities of your feelings as fully as you can. Be sensitive to your own experience. If your feelings or sensations do not match the feelings or sensations mentioned in the exercise description, do not be concerned; these descriptions are only indications of what you might feel. Bring your breath and your awareness to each feeling, and allow its special tones to permeate your body and mind.

As your feelings expand, you will become familiar with different stages of relaxation. Beginning an exercise, you may find that you are watching yourself do the exercise; there is a division between you and your sensations. As you continue to relax and explore a movement with light concentration, simultaneously breathing at an even level and expanding the sensations stimulated by this exercise, experience becomes richer and more substantial in quality; a feeling of 'the exercise doing itself' begins.

Each repetition of the exercise becomes an opportunity to explore more fully the feelings activated by the movement, a chance to bring body, mind, and senses together. Mental as well as physical energies contact one another and become integrated. Later, there may be no sense of 'self' at all, only ever-expanding awareness.

You may find that some of the exercises have an immediate effect; others may affect you gradually. Certain exercises may not seem to affect you at all, even after several practice sessions. If an exercise does not seem to generate much feeling or energy, you may be holding tension somewhere which blocks the flow of sensation. Perhaps you are holding a particular position too rigidly. Try moving slightly within the position; tension may relax and release a different quality of energy. If the exercise continues to have little effect, let it go for a while. Later you may return to an exercise you earlier set aside and find it effective.

Continue to explore your feelings in a sensitive way during the sitting period of each exercise. The sitting posture described in Part One, the seven gestures, encourages an even flow of feeling throughout your body. If you wish, sit before practicing as well. Sit and move within your feelings; develop a meditative awareness.

When you finish practicing, be sure to let your next activity also be a form of Kum Nye. Expand your feelings while eating, walking, or seeing. Let relaxation inform every experience, so your entire life becomes a part of an expanding, widening meditation.

Stage One

As you begin these exercises, remember to wear loose, comfortable clothing; tight clothes (especially clothes tight around the waist) will restrict your movement and distract you from the feelings generated by the exercise. Remove shoes, watches, jewelry, glasses, or contact lenses. If you eat beforehand, eat lightly, and wait for at least an hour after eating to begin practice.

Some of these exercises are done sitting, some are done standing. For the sitting exercises, you will need a mat or cushion so that your pelvis is higher than your legs. You may want to experiment with different ways of sitting and crossing your legs until you find the position that permits the most ease of movement. If sitting cross-legged is too uncomfortable for you, then sit in a straight chair with your feet flat on the floor.

Most of the exercises in this stage release tension in the upper body—the shoulders, chest, back, arms, neck, and head. As tension in these areas lessens, it is possible to feel more in the heart. These exercises develop valuable healing energies, so be sure to go deeply into some of them. You will find them most effective if you have already developed the massage and some of the exercises in Part One of this book.

Practice as regularly as you can. If you miss a day or so, do not be concerned; you will not lose ground.

Encourage yourself and continue to practice. When you are very busy, doing an exercise even for five or ten minutes on a break from work will have a beneficial effect.

At times you may find that you are unable to touch feelings during an exercise. This may indicate that your body and mind are too excited or tense to communicate well with each other. You may be so full of thoughts and images that you are unable to sense your feelings clearly. You may be too upset to breathe in the even and gentle way that awakens nurturing feelings. This unsteady state of mind will most likely cause your physical balance to be unsteady as well.

When you are feeling 'off balance', sit quietly for a while before exercising, and concentrate lightly on your breathing. Let your breath become light and soft. When you begin to feel more relaxed and calm, slowly begin an exercise. As relaxation deepens, a flowing, moving quality like waves may arise. The feeling may be smooth and flowing, almost magically sweet. With regular practice this feeling can be expanded. Relaxation will deepen, until you find that this flowing rhythm has passed into all of your daily activities.

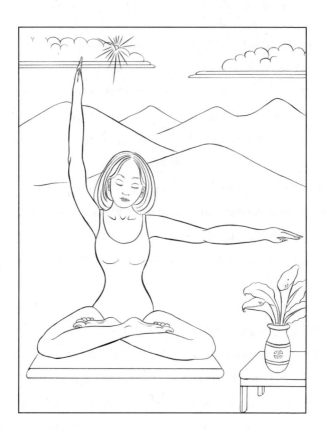

Exercise 35   Loosening up the Mind

If you are pregnant or have had any kind of neck injury, it is best not to do this exercise.

Sit cross-legged on a mat or cushion with your back straight. Slowly lift the arms away from your sides until they are stretched out at shoulder height, palms down. Close your eyes. Breathing softly through both nose and mouth, very slowly begin to rotate your head in clockwise direction. As you complete the rotation, also begin to rotate your right arm up, back, down, and forward. Coordinate the two circles, making them large and full.

This movement may seem awkward or even difficult at first, for we are not accustomed to moving our heads and arms in this way. Your mind may be set in old, familiar patterns of movement and holding that you feel unwilling to change.

Use the movement to 'exercise' the feeling of unwillingness until it changes into a natural flow of feeling and energy. Relax the belly and let your breath become even, connecting it with the movement, so the rotations become smooth and spacious.

Make three slow coordinated rotations of the head and right arm; then find a place in the movement where you can comfortably change the direction of the circles of both head and arm, and make three slow rotations in the other direction. Be sure to keep your left arm outstretched at shoulder height throughout; this will make the movement easier.

Go deeply into the sensations generated by the movement, unifying body, breath, and mind. You may feel delicious warmth in your arms and at the back of your neck. Let the warmth flow down your spine and spread throughout your body.

When you finish the rotations, slowly lower your hands to your knees. Rest for a few minutes, continuing to expand the feelings within and around your body.

Now repeat the above sequence of rotations with the head and the left arm. Rest afterward for a few minutes, breathing gently and evenly.

To complete the exercise, again do the whole series of rotations, but this time with the head and arm moving in opposite directions from each other: when the head moves clockwise, the arm will move forward, down, back, and up. Begin with your head and right arm, rest for a few minutes with your hands on your knees, and repeat the movement with the head and left arm.

Remember to keep your breathing soft and even, uniting it with your sensations. At the end, sit quietly for five to ten minutes, amplifying and extending your sensations and feelings.

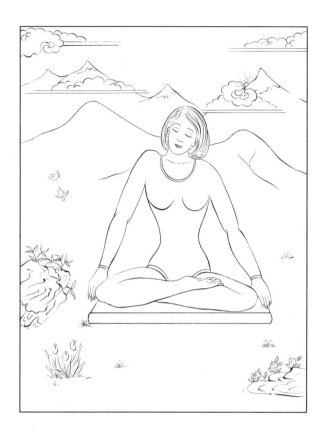

Exercise 36   Awakening the Senses

If you are pregnant or have had any kind of neck injury, it is best not to do this exercise.

Sit cross-legged on a mat or cushion with a straight back. Lift the arms away from your sides a few inches, with the palms facing behind you. Be sure your pelvis is high enough to allow your arms to move without your hands touching the floor. Gently close your eyes, and slowly begin to rotate your right shoulder up, back, down, and forward. Your right hand will also move in a circle. As you complete the first rotation, also begin head rotations in a clockwise direction. Coordinate the two movements, making the circles as full as you can. As you move, breathe gently through nose and mouth, and concentrate lightly on the back of your neck. Make three coordinated rotations, then change the direction of the rotations of both shoulder and head and continue three more times. After finishing, put the hands on the knees and rest briefly, allowing the feelings awakened by the slow rotations to flow down your spine and be distributed throughout your body.

Now in the same way as before, lift your arms away from your sides a few inches with the palms facing behind you, and very slowly rotate your left shoulder—up, back, down, and forward—coordinating the movement with a clockwise rotation of your head.

Make three rotations in this way; then gently change the direction of the rotations and repeat the movement three times. After completing these movements, bring your hands to your knees and rest for a few minutes, continuing to expand your sensations.

To complete this exercise, repeat the series of rotations, this time with the shoulder and head moving in opposite directions: when the shoulder moves up, back, down, and forward, the head will move counterclockwise. Begin with the right shoulder and head, rest for a few minutes with your hands on your knees, and repeat the movement with the left shoulder and head. Develop the shape of the movement, with special attention to high and low points (when the head is at its highest point in the movement, the shoulder is lowest, and vice versa), and the points when the head and shoulder are nearest and farthest apart from each other. Allow the feelings generated by the movement to permeate the shape until you experience a 'feeling-shape'.

Sit quietly in the sitting posture for five to ten minutes, enlarging and deepening the sensations within and around your body.

This exercise releases tension in the back of the neck, the shoulders, the upper back, and the lower back.

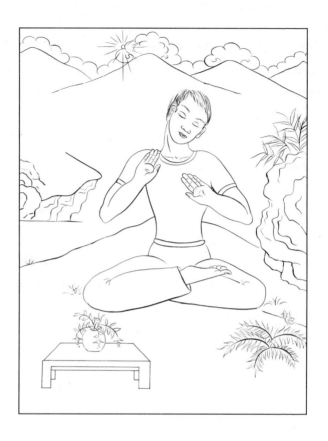

Exercise 37 Balancing the Senses

If you are pregnant or have had any kind of neck injury, it is best not to do this exercise.

Sit cross-legged on a mat or cushion with your back straight and your hands on your knees. Lift your arms in front of you to chest height with your elbows loosely bent and your hands relaxed, the palms down and the fingers pointing forward. Picture two large clock faces side by side, facing you. Imagine that your hand is at three on the left clock face, and your right hand is at nine on the right clock face. Your hands will be a few inches apart.

Now at the same time, very slowly, draw two large clockwise circles with your hands and arms, beginning at three and moving toward six with the left hand, beginning at nine and moving toward twelve with the right hand. Make the circles as large as possible without overlapping them.

When you have this movement going in a smooth rhythm, add to it a very slow clockwise rotation of your head, with your eyes closed. Coordinate and balance the three simultaneous movements, keeping your belly relaxed and your breathing very soft and smooth, through both nose and mouth. Continue for two minutes, then slowly diminish the movement until you no longer move at all. Lower the hands to the knees, sit for two minutes, expanding the sensations stimulated by these circling movements.

Now repeat the exercise, this time making counter-clockwise circles with both the arms and the head (move the left hand from three toward twelve on the left clock face, and the right hand from nine toward six on the right clock face). Continue for two minutes, then sit quietly for five minutes, continuing to extend the sensations within and around your body. When you can balance your body and mind in coordinating three different movements at the same time, the senses become balanced as well, and sensations will arise within that balance.

Exercise 38   Enjoying Sensation

Stand well balanced with your feet a few inches apart, back straight, and arms relaxed at the sides. Breathing gently and evenly through both nose and mouth, with the belly relaxed, loosely and vigorously shake your shoulders in any way you wish. Relax the back of your neck, and concentrate lightly there, letting your head hang. Your torso and lower body remain still. Continue for three minutes, shaking out tightness. Then sit in the sitting posture for five minutes, expanding the sensations generated, distributing them through the body.

You may feel a deep, warm sensation in the back of your neck flowing down your spine, and perhaps spreading to your chest and arms. The flow of feeling through the neck to the head may be more free.

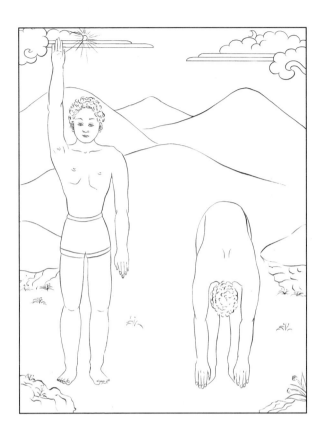

Exercise 39   Swimming in Space

Stand well balanced with your feet a comfortable distance apart, your back straight, and your arms stretched out in front of you at shoulder height, palms down. Breathing through both nose and mouth, with your belly relaxed, you simultaneously move one arm up and the other arm down, keeping the arms and hands straight and relaxed.

Move very slowly. At first do not move the arms very far—then gradually extend the movement until finally each arm moves up and down as far as it can go. At the furthest points of the movement, relax the back of the neck and head. Pay attention to the particular sense of space awakened by this exercise; you may feel a quality like swimming.

Continue the full movement of the arms for three to five minutes. Then slowly begin to decrease the range of the movement until your arms are still, and extended in front of you at shoulder height. Slowly lower them to your sides, and stand quietly for a few minutes, expanding your sensations and feelings.

Now slowly lift your arms in front of you until they are overhead with the palms facing forward. Keep the arms parallel to each other and straight. Moving arms, head, and torso together, bend down from the waist until your fingers almost touch the floor; then swing up slowly until your back is straight and your arms are outstretched overhead.

Continue this slow swinging movement, down and up, three or nine times. Be sure to keep the arms straight throughout the movement. To complete the exercise, lower your arms to your sides from the overhead position, and sit in the sitting posture for five to ten minutes, expanding the sensations quickened by this movement.

The first part of this exercise releases tension in the back, the throat, the neck, and the back of the head. The second part distributes the feelings released in the first part of the exercise throughout the whole body.

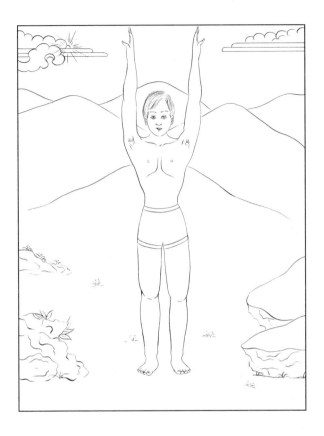

Exercise 40   Awareness of the Senses

This exercise differs from the preceding exercise in the position of the hands and arms. Stand well balanced with your feet a comfortable distance apart, back straight, and the arms relaxed at the sides.

Turn your hands inward so the palms face out to the sides, and stick out your thumbs so they also point out to the side. With the hands in this position, slowly lift the arms in front of you to shoulder height. Breathe easily through both nose and mouth simultaneously, and keep the belly soft and relaxed.

Now, keeping your arms straight but relaxed, begin to move one arm up and the other arm down. Move them just a short distance at first, concentrating on the feelings in and around them as they move slowly through space. Gradually, as your feelings expand, extend the range of movement and the space through which your arms pass until both arms are moving up and down as far as they will go. Expand fully the special qualities of feeling stimulated by this movement, keeping your belly relaxed and your breathing soft, even, and slow.

Continue for three to five minutes, then decrease the range of the movement until your arms are still, outstretched in front of you at shoulder height. Slowly lower them to your sides, relax your hands, and stand quietly for a few minutes, expanding the feelings.

Once again turn your hands inward until the palms face out to your sides, and stick out your thumbs so they also point out to the side. With your hands in this position, slowly lift your arms in front of you until they are overhead, keeping them parallel to each other and straight. Then bend forward slowly from the waist until your fingers almost touch the floor.

Let your head hang loosely between your arms. Relax your belly and breathe easily through both nose and mouth. Then slowly rise with your head between your outstretched arms until you stand upright with your arms overhead. Continue to bend and rise slowly three times, sensing deeply the spatial quality stimulated by this position of the hands and arms.

Slowly begin to move slightly faster, swinging up and down, letting your feelings merge with the rhythm of your body. As you move faster, make sure that your belly stays relaxed, and your movement and breathing are smooth and even. If you begin to lose touch with the feeling quality of the movement, slow down until the sensations become stronger; then slowly build up more speed. Swing up and down nine more times. You may feel a special tingling sensation in your arms.

From the upright position, lower your arms to your sides, relax your hands, and stand quietly for a minute. Then sit in the sitting posture for five to ten minutes, breathing gently and evenly. Allow the sensations to be distributed throughout the body and expand beyond the body to the surrounding universe.

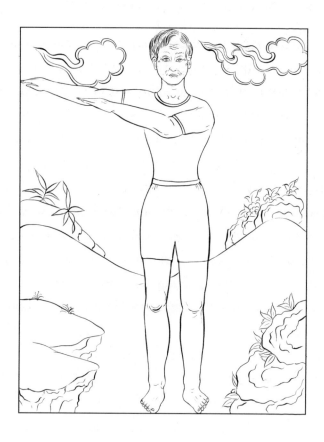

Exercise 41   Body Alertness

Stand facing forward with your feet a few inches apart,
your back straight, and your arms relaxed at your sides.
Inhale through both nose and mouth, and slowly raise
your arms in front of you to shoulder height, palms down.
Keep your head and chest very still.

As you exhale, very gradually move both arms to the
right as far as possible, keeping the rest of the body and
especially the chest, relaxed and still. Lead the movement

with your right arm. The right arm will be straight and the left arm will bend slightly at the elbow.

Now while inhaling, let your arms come back very slowly to the front. Without stopping, continue moving to the left while exhaling. Lead the movement to the left with the left arm; the left arm will be straight and the right arm bent slightly at the elbow. Throughout the movement, your belly should be relaxed and your body straight and well balanced.

Do the complete movement, once to each side, three or nine times. Then sit in the sitting posture for five to ten minutes with the feelings awakened by the exercise.

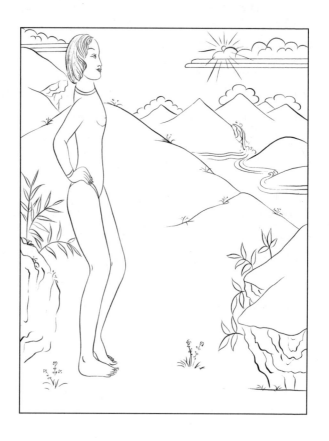

Exercise 42 Balancing the Body

Do this exercise barefoot. Stand well balanced with your
hands on your hips, your feet a few inches apart, your back
straight, and your chest high. Breathe gently through both
nose and mouth. Slowly lift your right heel so your right
toes and your left foot carry your weight. Now in a slow,
continuous motion, with both feet always in contact with
the floor, lower your right heel to the floor and simultaneously lift your left heel. Continue in a slow, smooth

rhythm, lifting the heel of one foot while lowering the heel of the other to the floor. Your weight and balance will be primarily on the toes and balls of the feet.

Notice the point at which you are standing on the toes of both feet, as one heel moves up and the other moves down. Intensify the 'high' at this point by stretching up on the toes. Then intensify the 'low' as well: as your heel comes back to the floor, push the hip on that side of your body back and down as if sitting down in a low chair, bending both knees. Keep your back straight. Notice the change in feeling-tone as the vertical range of the movement increases.

Continue this movement until it is no longer jerky or unbalanced and both the breath and the movement are slow and smooth. Then (but not before) do the movement a little faster, but not so fast that you lose touch with the feeling-tone. Finally, slow down the movement until it stops. Sit for five to ten minutes, expanding the sensations stimulated in your body, mind, and senses. This exercise balances the body and stimulates energy in the toe, knee, thigh, and hip joints.

Exercise 43   Sensing Body Energy

Stand well balanced with your feet a comfortable distance apart and your arms relaxed at your sides. Closing your eyes, take a few moments to relax and sense your inner experience. What is your emotional state? Are you feeling calm, restless, tired? Is your mind filled with thoughts?

Now very slowly open your eyes, and begin to move spontaneously in any way that feels relaxing. Breathe gently through both nose and mouth, and relax your belly. Perhaps make swinging or rotating motions, or gently twist, rock, bend, or sway. Let the feeling of relaxation guide and balance your movement. Allow the relaxed feeling to spread everywhere in your body—to your jaw, neck, shoulders, upper back, arms, elbows, wrists, fingers, middle back, lower back, pelvis, thighs, knees, ankles, and toes. Be attentive to every joint, every muscle and bone. Feel free to do any movement that increases the feeling of relaxation. Continue for five minutes or more.

Now slowly develop a different quality of movement—a short, fast, light motion. This is not a heavy motion like kicking, but more like a rhythmical shaking. Perhaps begin the movement in your legs and hands, and then allow it to spread to more and more of your body, until finally your whole body participates in the movement. When you find a tense spot, let the shaking gently open it up. Continue for several minutes, and then sit in the seven gestures for at least five to ten minutes with the feelings stimulated by the movement.

Stage Two

The exercises continue to release tension in the upper body, balancing inner energies so that feeling can flow more freely, and body and mind can make contact with one another. Exercises 52 and 55 energize the lower body.

Some of these exercises involve holding a position for a period of time. You may wish to measure the time by counting your outbreaths. Before beginning the exercise, time your breathing for a few minutes, and calculate your average number of outbreaths per minute.

When you release tension after holding, do so very slowly and gradually. When the process of releasing tension is slow, awareness of energy increases, and it is easier to continue the feelings and distribute them to your whole body. Quick release would cut off the feelings of stimulation and exhilaration.

Fully explore each exercise you select to practice until you become familiar with the range of feelings it stimulates and its special qualities of balance. Do not go too fast or try to do too much. If you begin to feel overwhelmed by the possibilities opening up to you in these exercises, stay with that feeling and bring it into your practice. Let your self-imposed limitations open into deeper feeling and sensation; allow yourself to be larger and larger until you see that all limitations are arbitrary and self-imposed, and your experience can be as large as the universe itself.

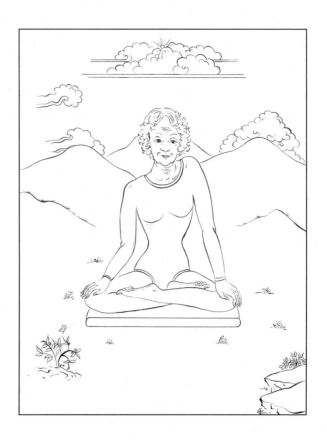

Exercise 44   Touching the Senses

Sit cross-legged on a mat or cushion with your hands on your knees and your back straight. In a continuous, coordinated movement, alternately rotate your shoulders from front to back, as if back-pedaling a bicycle. Move them quickly, a little roughly. Let your shoulders be very loose as you do this, and your head still. Picture the spine and the spaces between the vertebrae being massaged by the action of the shoulder blades. Continue for one minute.

Now gradually change the quality of the movement so it becomes gentler, longer and slower, more soothing and massage-like in quality. Let this massage stimulate your senses, relieving tension and awakening sensation even between layers of skin and muscle tissue. Sensations may also be quickened in the heart center, awakening perhaps a feeling of yearning. Continue this massage for three to five minutes and then sit quietly for an equal amount of time, expanding the feeling-tone developed by this exercise.

• To explore this exercise further, try this variation. Rotate the left shoulder front to back twenty-one times. Repeat with your right shoulder. Sit for several minutes, experiencing the sensations stimulated by the movement. Again rotate your left shoulder as before, twenty-one times, now more slowly. Repeat with your right shoulder. Sit for two minutes, experiencing the sensations stimulated by the movement.

Again rotate your left shoulder as before, twenty-one times, this time more slowly. Repeat with your right shoulder. Then sit with your feelings for two minutes.

Repeat the movement, first with the left, then with the right shoulder, this time even more slowly. Then sit for five minutes with the feelings and sensations that have emerged from the movement.

These exercises can also be done standing.

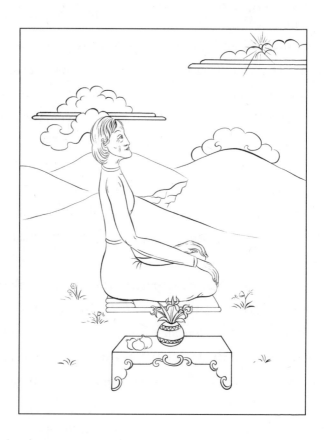

Exercise 45   Balancing Inner Energy

It is best not to do this exercise if you are pregnant. If you have had a neck or back injury, or an operation within three or four months, do it mindfully.

In this exercise you will make a circle in front of your body with your chin. Sit cross-legged on a mat or cushion with your hands relaxed on your knees, and breathe gently through both nose and mouth. Slowly jut and stretch your chin directly forward as far as possible. Do not be afraid to stretch strenuously (unless you have had a neck or back injury; then do this extremely sensitively). Be sure that the chest and neck remain straight and only the jaw and chin move forward; the movement then has great strength and energy and leads to a certain quality of relaxation.

Maintaining the strenuous stretch and breathing very, very softly through both nose and mouth, slowly move your chin down toward your chest. When your chin nears your chest, slowly draw it in as close as possible to your neck. The muscles of the back of your neck will become very tense and strong, and may shimmy a little. Maintain this quality of strength in the neck muscles, relax your hands and belly, and continuing the circle, slowly lift the chin up as far as you can, separating the muscles of your neck and shoulders. Then slowly jut your chin forward to complete the circle.

Release the tension very slowly, so you are aware of subtle qualities of feeling, and sit quietly for a few minutes, breathing gently and expanding the sensations in your body. Repeat the movement twice more. Sit for a few minutes after each repetition, and for five to ten minutes at the end, sensing and expanding the feelings generated by this movement.

It is important to loosen the neck muscles after this balancing exercise. Breathing softly and gently, move your head forward and back, turn it from side to side, and bend it laterally (so your ear moves toward of your shoulder).

Be sure to do these neck stretches every time you finish this exercise. You may also want to massage the neck muscles.

On first glance, this exercise may not seem appealing. It entails performing a motion—jutting out the chin and drawing it back—that may look or sound unattractive. It is also a motion that the body does not ordinarily perform. However, when you try this exercise several times, you may find that it is very effective in releasing tension in the neck area, and that it elicits unusually relaxing feelings. Try it not only during your daily practice, but also during times when you are especially tired or tense.

This exercise releases tension in the neck, head, shoulders, chest, and spine, and equalizes and balances all the energies in these areas.

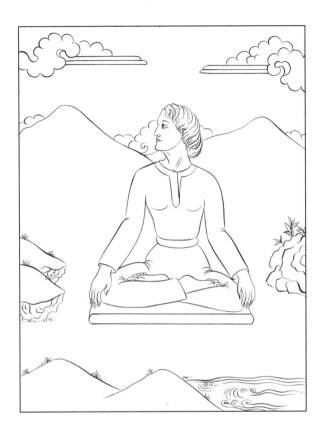

Exercise 46   Refreshing Energy

It is best not to do this exercise if you are pregnant. If you have had a neck or back injury, or an operation within three or four months, do it mindfully.

In this exercise your chin will trace a path like two half circles side by side, similar to an 'm'. Sit cross-legged on a mat or cushion, with your hands on your knees. Breathe softly through both nose and mouth. Slowly jut your chin forward, using some strength. Your chest remains straight.

In this position, slowly let your chin draw an arc up and to the right. As your chin approaches your right shoulder, look up to the ceiling. When your chin is over your right shoulder, slowly lower it toward the shoulder, while continuing to look up. Keep your shoulders back a little and loosen your stomach. With your chin still over your shoulder, slowly lift your chin toward the ceiling, and slowly retrace the arc just drawn, moving from right to left. When you face straight ahead, slowly arch your chin down toward your chest.

Now, without stopping, repeat the above movement, this time to the left side. When you finish, very slowly lift your chin from your chest, releasing the tension and sensing the qualities of feeling stimulated by the exercise. Sit for a few minutes before repeating the exercise.

Do the exercise very slowly three or nine times, sitting briefly after each repetition. At the end, sit for five to ten minutes, allowing the feelings stimulated by the movement to expand.

Afterward, gently loosen the neck muscles in three ways: move your head forward and back, from side to side, and so that your ear moves toward your shoulder. Be sure to do this each time you finish the exercise. Also massage your neck gently if you wish.

Like the preceding exercise, this exercise releases tension in the neck, head, shoulders, chest, and spine, and equalizes energies in these areas.

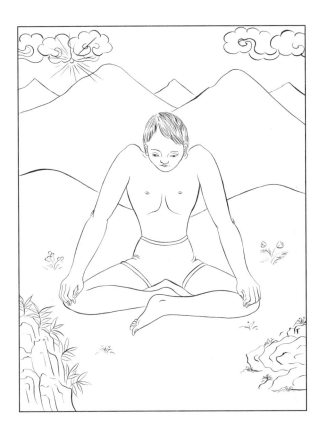

Exercise 47 Integrating Body and Mind

It is best not to do this exercise if you are pregnant. Do it gently if you have had a neck or back injury or an operation within three or four months.

Sit on a mat or cushion with your legs loosely crossed. It is important to have both feet rest on the mat or the floor. Place your hands on your knees, lift your shoulders a little, and proceed to move them backward slightly so your arms straighten.

Slowly jut your jaw forward, using some strength, but being sure not to stretch too much. Then, breathing very softly through both nose and mouth, slowly arch your chin down toward your chest. Hold this position for one to three minutes, keeping the breath light and even.

Then slowly lift your chin, and very slowly release the tension in your jaw, shoulders, and neck, sensing the subtle qualities of feeling that arise. Let these feelings be distributed throughout your body.

Rest for a few minutes, then repeat the exercise two more times, resting for several minutes after each repetition and for five to ten minutes at the end.

Each time you finish the exercise, gently loosen the neck muscles. Slowly move your head forward and back, from side to side, and so that your ear moves toward your shoulder. Also massage your neck gently if you wish.

Like the two preceding exercises, this exercise releases tension in the neck, head, shoulders, chest, and spine, and balances their interconnecting energies.

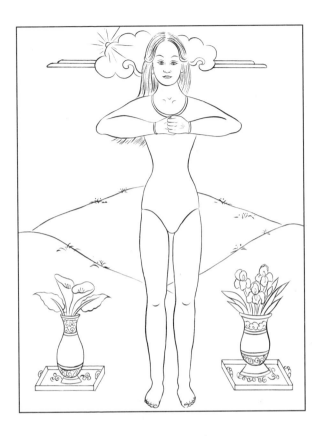

Exercise 48   Enjoying Space

Stand well balanced with your feet a few inches apart, back straight, and arms relaxed at your sides. Breathe evenly through nose and mouth. Bring the elbows and hands to the level of the heart, hook the fingers together and pull tensely as if to draw the hands apart. (Your fingernails must be short!) Move your shoulders back a little.

Facing forward with your eyes soft and still, your feet firmly planted on the ground, and your knees straight but not locked, very slowly twist to the right as far as you can. Take about one minute for this movement. Then gradually return to the front and without stopping twist slowly to the left.

Throughout the entire movement, keep your belly and hips relaxed and your breath easy, while maintaining the tension in hands, arms, and shoulders. Then unhurriedly return to the front and very slowly release the tension, going deeply into the sensations awakened in your body, especially in your spine and shoulders. Slowly lower your arms to your sides, and rest briefly in either a standing or sitting position, continuing to expand the sensations in your body.

Do the complete movement, once to each side, three times, resting for a few minutes after each repetition and sitting for five to ten minutes at the end.

This exercise can also be done sitting.

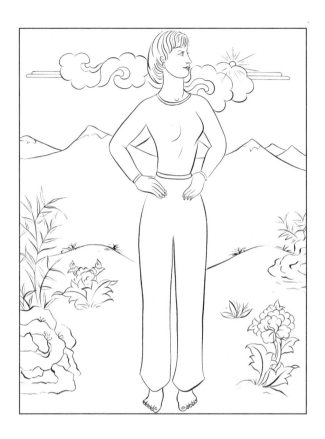

Exercise 49   Exercising in Space

Stand with your feet a comfortable distance apart, your back straight, and your body balanced. Breathe lightly and evenly through both nose and mouth. Place your hands on your hips, with as much contact as possible between them. Plant your legs and feet firmly and straighten your knees without locking them.

In this position, very slowly twist only your upper body to the right, moving the head and eyes with the shoulders, arms, and chest. Keep your elbows out and use your hands to help keep the pelvis still by pushing forward on the right hip and backward on the left hip. Take about thirty seconds for this movement. Then slowly return to the front, again pushing your hands against your hips to keep the pelvis still, and continue turning your upper body to the left.

Your pelvis may move slightly, but if it moves more than a very little, stop and begin again. You may find it helpful to first twist the torso a few times while facing forward, and then add the movement of the head. As you continue to practice the exercise, you will learn to differentiate the turning of the upper body from the turning of the lower body. While the upper body gently exercises, the lower body is steady and rooted, with a strong, concentrative quality. These two qualities give the body a particular kind of balance.

Do the complete movement, to the right and to the left, three or nine times. Then sit in the sitting posture for five minutes, sensing the special character of the energy generated by this movement.

This exercise releases muscular tension in the chest, the upper and middle back, and the neck, and also relaxes the stomach.

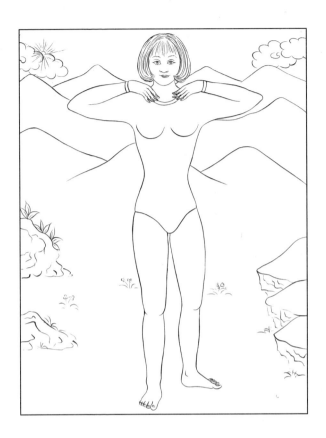

Exercise 50   Interacting Body and Mind

Stand well balanced with your legs a comfortable distance apart, the back straight, and the arms relaxed at your sides. Turn your left foot so the toes point to the left and place your right foot about twelve inches in front of you, with the toes pointing forward and the heel on a line with the heel of the left foot. Lift your arms away from your sides to shoulder height, and place your hands on your shoulders so the fingers are on the front of the shoulders and

251

the thumbs are on the back. Press with as much contact between hand and shoulder as possible.

In this position, with your eyes open, begin to rotate your upper torso. Leading with your left elbow, turn your torso to the left as far as you can go without straining, then bend down to the side, letting your head hang. Without stopping, and without raising your torso, continue rotating to the right, and then slowly straighten up on your right side. As you come up, look toward the ceiling. Then again, leading with the left elbow, slowly turn your torso to the left and begin another rotation. Breathe easily through both nose and mouth throughout, and continue to press your hands against your shoulders.

Do three or nine rotations, very slowly. Then reverse the position of your feet, so the right foot points to the right, and the left foot is about twelve inches in front of you, with the toes pointing forward. In this position, do three or nine very slow rotations, leading the turning of the torso with the right elbow. When you finish, sit for five to ten minutes, expanding the sensations stimulated by this movement.

This exercise relieves headache, and also relieves tension in the back, shoulders, and legs.

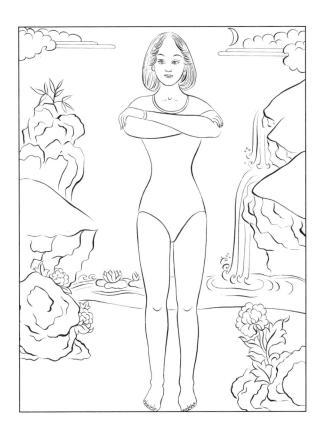

Exercise 51   Touching Alertness

This exercise will be most effective if you have already released tension in your back and neck through massage and some of the exercises in Stage One.

Stand in a well-balanced way with your feet a comfortable distance apart and your back straight. Unhurriedly lift your arms to shoulder height, cross them in front with the elbows at shoulder level, and lightly hold the opposite arm just above the elbow. The arm bones should be well balanced in the shoulder socket, not too far forward nor too far back.

Look straight ahead, and thrust your crossed arms twice to the right, beginning the second thrust where the first thrust ends. Exhale through both nose and mouth as fully as possible with each thrust.

With each thrust, increase the distance of the movement until the second thrust brings your arms to the right as far as they can go. Only the arms and shoulders move; the head and torso remain still. You may hear cracking in your middle back, or the back of your neck, as muscles along the spine are adjusted. These movements and breath should have a strong impulse, yet not be shocking or tense. Move easily, in a natural way.

After the thrusts, slowly return your arms to the front, and inhale slowly and fully. Now loosen your shoulders, back muscles, and belly, and do the movement to the left. Do the complete movement, once to the right and once to the left, three times. Then sit in the sitting posture for five minutes or more, following the sensations and feelings quickened in your body.

This exercise relieves tension in the shoulders and the middle back. Through the exhalations, any holding in the lower body is also released.

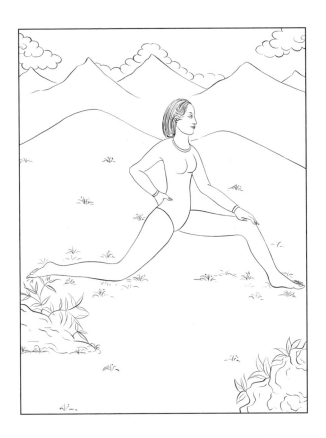

Exercise 52 Vitalizing Energy

Kneel on your right knee with the toes pointing behind you; bend the left knee and place your left foot on the floor as far in front of you as possible. Place your right hand on your right hip and your left hand on your left knee. Face forward with your back straight, and in this position, keeping your left foot in the same place, shift your weight forward and increase the bend in your left knee until you feel a stretch in both thighs. Make sure the legs are wide apart.

Relax both arms, hands and the chest, and hold the position for about thirty seconds, breathing gently through both nose and mouth and feeling the sensations produced by the stretch.

Then very slowly shift your weight back onto your right leg, straighten your left leg, and flex the left ankle so the toes point to the ceiling. Attend to the subtle qualities of feeling that arise as you do this leg stretch. Then gradually relax the left leg and foot and kneel on both knees. Rest briefly, continuing to feel the sensations stimulated by the stretches.

Now reverse the position of the legs and hands so you kneel on your left knee and stand on your right foot, with your right hand on your right knee and your left hand on your left hip. Repeat the exercise in this position.

Do the complete exercise, first on one side, then on the other, three times, resting briefly after each repetition. At the end, sit in the sitting posture for five to ten minutes, expanding the feelings quickened by this exercise.

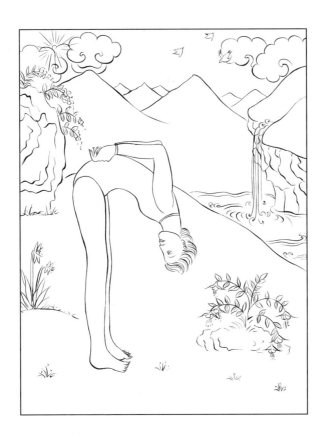

Exercise 53   Balancing Energy

Stand with your feet a comfortable distance apart. Put your hands behind your back, interlacing the fingers so they are on the same side as the palms. Bend forward slowly from the waist, and use your lowest knuckles to massage the big muscles alongside the spine. (This massage can be done through clothes, but is best done directly on the skin.)

Stay down, and let your body be very relaxed as you continue to massage slowly. Be sure to let your head hang loosely from your neck. This massage can be done at different tempos, and with different degrees of pressure. You may wish to start at the lower region of the spine and slowly rub in one spot until the tension begins to loosen. Then move slowly up the spine, pausing to rub whenever your knuckles touch upon sensitive muscles. Continue up the spine as far as you can reach.

When you finish, relax your arms and rise very slowly, breathing gently, carrying your weight in your legs. Then stand quietly for a few minutes.

This exercise relieves tension, balances the breath, and encourages an even flow of energy throughout the body. It is especially useful after heavy exercise, or after exercising the lower body. Once is usually enough.

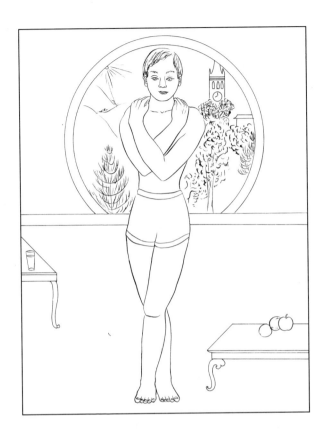

Exercise 54   Loosening up the Self-Image

Stand well balanced with your back straight and your arms
relaxed at your sides. Cross your arms in front of your
chest, the right over the left, and hold your shoulders with
your hands, letting the elbows hang down. Cross the right
leg over the left and place your right foot next to the left
foot. In this position, breathing gently through both nose
and mouth, very slowly bend forward from the waist as
low as possible without straining, letting your head hang.

Then very slowly rise up and arch backward slightly, concentrating on your feet.

Do the movement three or nine times in this position; then cross the left arm over the right, and the left leg over the right, and repeat the exercise three or nine times. Notice the different qualities of feeling stimulated by the change in position. Then sit in the sitting posture for five to ten minutes, expanding the sensations stimulated by this movement.

If you want to extend this exercise, try it three times with the legs crossed left over right and the arms crossed right over left. Then reverse the position of both arms and legs and repeat three more times. Then sit for five to ten minutes, expanding sensations and feelings.

• As a variation of this exercise, stand with the feet spread wide apart, and cross your arms behind your back, holding your forearms just above the elbows. In this position, very slowly bend forward from the waist, letting your head hang. Very slowly rise and bend backward slightly. Repeat the movement three or nine times, then sit in the sitting posture for five to ten minutes, expanding the feelings quickened by this version of the movement. These exercises stimulate the skin and activate new mental and muscular patterns.

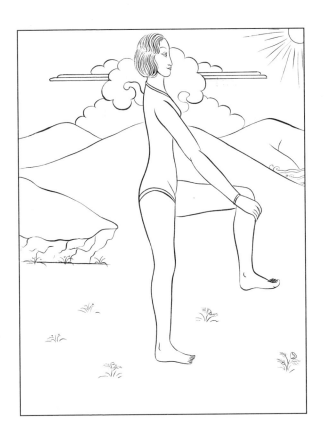

Exercise 55   Balancing Mind and Senses

Stand barefoot on the floor or ground with your feet a few inches apart, your back straight, your arms at your sides, and the body balanced. Slowly bend the left knee, clasp it with interlaced hands, draw it up toward your chest, and flex your left ankle so the toes point toward the ceiling. Relax your pelvis and move your shoulders backward a little. Look straight ahead with soft eyes, and balance in this position for one to three minutes, in a relaxed and even casual way, breathing gently through both nose and mouth. At first hold your leg tightly with your hands, then slowly release the holding (without moving the leg) until your hands become relaxed. As you do this, keep your chest as relaxed as possible.

Now, keeping your hands around your knee, slowly lower your left leg to the point where you feel control of the movement can pass easily to your leg. Then open your hands gently and casually and lower your leg to the ground. By sensing the moments at which certain muscles take over a movement, we can learn to combine relaxation and controlled movement. During each phase—lifting the leg, holding the position, lowering the leg, and releasing the hands—let your attitude be casual and unambitious. Then you can be sensitive to subtle muscular and energetic changes.

Slowly bring your left foot to the floor, and notice the special feeling-tones that arise just before the foot touches the ground. Continue the exercise, lifting the right knee and balancing on the left leg. Do the complete movement (first one side, then the other) three or nine times, and then sit for five to ten minutes, expanding the feelings that were quickened by this exercise.

This exercise stimulates different kinds of energy in the lower body.

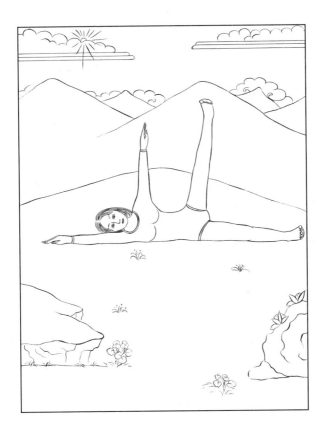

Exercise 56   Coordinating Body and Mind

Lie on your right side, your left leg on top of the right, with your right arm extended overhead on the floor, palm down. Rest your head on your right arm, and place your left arm along the side of your body, palm down. Make sure your body is lying in a straight line.

Keeping your legs straight, flex both ankles so your toes point toward your head. Slowly stretch both your left arm and leg as if to lengthen them. Then, continuing the stretch, lift your left arm and leg until the arm is vertical and the leg is as high as it can comfortably go. Keep the ankles flexed. Breathing gently and evenly through both nose and mouth, coordinate the movement so both the arm and leg slowly cover the distance in the same amount of time.

Then, moving as slowly as you can, so you feel more, gently lower both your arm and leg, while continuing the stretch. Relax and rest a minute, then repeat the movement two times, resting after each repetition. Then roll onto your left side and do the movement three more times, resting after each repetition.

At the end, roll onto your back and rest for five to ten minutes. Use the resting time to go deeper into the sensations activated by the movement.

Stage Three

The exercises in this group are a little more difficult than those in the earlier stages. This does not necessarily mean that the movements of the exercises are physically more difficult to do (although some of the movements are more demanding physically than those in earlier exercises). Rather, it means that greater concentration is needed to touch and develop the feeling-tones of the exercises.

After several months of practicing Kum Nye yoga, you will probably find that you are ready for some of these exercises. If you get little result from an exercise, however, put it aside for a while and come back to it later. The exercises toward the end of this stage should be left until you have quite a thorough experience of Kum Nye.

When you have made yourself entirely familiar with certain exercises, (including those in Stage One or Stage Two), try doing them for longer periods of time, perhaps as long as an hour. You might also want to begin experimenting with different tempos and different degrees of tension.

Try an exercise slowly; then very slowly; then do it faster, etcetera, and notice the different qualities of feeling at different speeds. All of the exercises done tensely can also be done 'loosely', and exercises done 'loosely' can also be done tensely. You might also want to try practicing at different times and in different places.

In many of these exercises, a certain position is held for a period of time. (Counting out breaths will help to measure the time.) Explore the quality of your holding, letting it be as relaxed as possible, without any special purpose. Remember to release the holding very slowly, so that you will feel more, and the sensations quickened by the exercise will last as long as possible. The longer a feeling-tone is expanded, the more it can spread beyond the body, stimulating interactions with surrounding 'space'.

As the feeling expands, bring breath, motion, feeling, and mind into a unity. Balance the breath, balance the senses, balance your awareness, balance your body. Then you develop a quality in your practice that is without holding or clinging, and you discover the joy of exercising without effort.

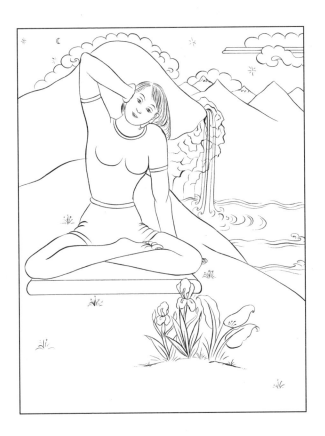

Exercise 57   Opening the Heart

Sit cross-legged on a mat or cushion and support yourself
with your right hand on the floor a comfortable distance
from you. Make sure your hand is not too far in front
or back. Place your left hand over the left ear, with the
elbow up. In this position, slowly arch to the right, keeping your right arm straight. Support yourself well with
your right hand so the arching of your left side can be
both maximized and balanced. Keep your knees down

as much as possible. Let your ribs lift away from your pelvis and open like a fan all the way to the underarm; let space expand within the bones of your hip and ribs, and in the muscles under your arm. Hold this position for one to three minutes, breathing softly and evenly through both nose and mouth.

Release the stretch very slowly—take about one minute for this—feeling the sensations generated by holding this position. Place your right hand over your right ear, supporting yourself with your left hand on the floor beside you, and arch slowly to the left. Do the complete exercise (first one side and then the other) three or nine times, then sit quietly in the sitting posture for five to ten minutes and taste the quality of this feeling of relaxation.

This exercise opens the heart center, improves breathing and circulation, and massages internal muscles.

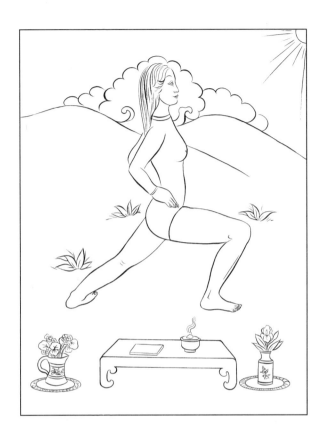

Exercise 58   Coordinating the Wholeness of Energy

Stand barefoot with your back straight, your feet wide
apart and pointed straight ahead, and your hands on your
hips. Your body and mind should be well-balanced and
concentrated. Turn your right foot to the right until it is
at a right angle to your left foot, bend your right knee, and
turn your torso to the right so you face the same direction as your right foot. Keep your left leg and your back
straight. Look at a spot on the wall in front of you near

the ceiling, with your head back, your chin in, your chest high, and your elbows out. Relax your belly and breathe smoothly through both nose and mouth.

In this position, lower your body by increasing the bend in your right knee and relaxing your pelvis. As you move down, keep your back and your left leg straight. Lower until you reach a place of both tension and energy. Do not worry if you are unable to find this place immediately; see how you feel at different points as you go down, and let your feelings guide you to the place where sensation is strongest.

When you find this place, remain there until you begin to shake; then return slowly to an upright position. Turn your right toes and torso to the left so you again face forward, and move your feet closer together. Move slowly and keep in contact with your feelings throughout the movement. Breathe softly and evenly so that all of the different steps involved in the exercise can flow smoothly and easily into each other.

If you find holding difficult to do at first, move down and up slowly several times until you become more familiar with the sensation of tension in the right knee and leg. Then try holding the position for a few seconds.

Now carefully change the position of your feet so that eventually your left foot points to the left and is at a right angle to your right foot. Continue the exercise on the left side. As you are moving, always take care to keep the movements flowing smoothly. Keep in touch with your feelings; do not let the movement become mechanical. Do the complete exercise, including both sides, three times, then sit in the sitting posture for five to ten minutes, expanding the feelings generated by this movement.

When you have practiced the above exercise ten times over a period of at least a week, try these variations.

• Coordinate your breathing with the exercise described above by slowly exhaling as you turn to the right and lower your body, and inhaling as you rise and return to the front. Exhale again slowly as you continue the exercise to the left. Do the motion very slowly and with concentration. There is one slow continuous stretch-motion and breath.

Always remain balanced. If you feel at any moment that you might lose control of the movement, then slowly bring your feet together and begin again with your legs a little closer together. Do the complete movement (to both right and left) three times; then sit for five to ten minutes, expanding your feelings. Through this exercise you can explore with clarity the interconnections among body, breath, and mind.

• Lower your body to the position described above, with your right foot turned to the right, at a right angle to your left foot, your right knee bent, your head and torso facing right, and your hands on your hips. Hold briefly, breathing very gently through both nose and mouth. Then, without returning to an upright position, very slowly rotate to the left—first turning your head to the left, then your shoulders, chest, pelvis, and feet. At the end of the rotation, your left foot will point to the left at a right angle to your right foot, and your head and torso will face the same direction as your left foot.

The rotation should be done extremely slowly, with a clear sense of controlling the movement. Be sure not to stretch too much. Continue holding the posture without returning to an upright position until you have done the complete movement (to both right and left) three times. Then slowly bring your feet together and sit in the sitting posture for ten minutes, expanding the energies generated by the exercise.

These exercises increase coordination. They develop the muscles of the legs and stimulate the flow of energy from the legs through the back and to the head.

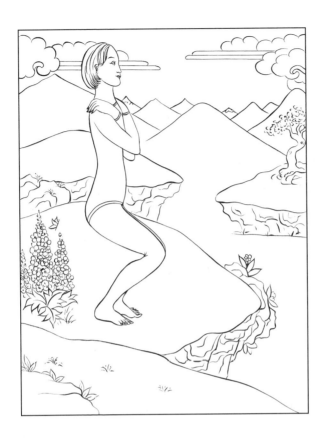

Exercise 59   Transforming Emotions

Stand well balanced with your feet close together and your
back straight. Cross your arms in front of your chest and
hold your shoulders with your hands, your elbows down.
With your legs together and your heels on the floor, bend
at the knees with your back straight, as if sitting down in a
low chair. Maintain internal balance as you lower, without
tensing up. When you have gone down a certain distance
in this position, you may find that tightness somewhere

prevents you from going further, and you are beginning to lift your heels from the floor. Stop and locate the tension—it may be in your pelvis or legs. Let it go, and continue to lower, keeping your back straight.

Well above a squatting position, you will discover a special place of balance and energy. You may need to move up and down a little until you find the right place. You may feel heat rise in your body, and you may begin to shake. You will feel pressure on your knees. Stay with these sensations and hold this position for one to five minutes, with your chin in and your back straight, concentrating on the energy in your spine.

Then very slowly return to a standing position, releasing the tension. Stand silently with your arms at your sides for three to five minutes; then repeat the exercise twice, standing or sitting quietly after each repetition. Now sit in the sitting posture for ten to fifteen minutes, expanding the sensations generated by this movement.

The close connections among our bodies, senses, and emotions allow us to affect our whole state of balance through a specific physical posture. Usually our emotions tend to throw us off balance. In this exercise, we can transform strong emotions such as resentment or anxiety, using the energy of the emotion to keep us balanced, rather than dissipating it through negativity. If you hold the position long enough, pure energy will flow throughout your body.

As you do the exercise, search out the inner tensions that throw you of balance and release them. Feel for any memory that makes you tense and relax it so that it flows like liquid. Breathe softly and gently into places of blockage. Even if an emotion is so strong that the holding manifests as pain, breathe into the pain until the holding relaxes and you discover a kernel of new energy. Keep your belly relaxed so that energy rising up from the legs can flow through your spine and be distributed to your whole body. Close your eyes and go inside for your inner balance. With practice, the exercise may become effortless.

This exercise stimulates all energies in the lower body, helps to stimulate hormones, and increases circulation.

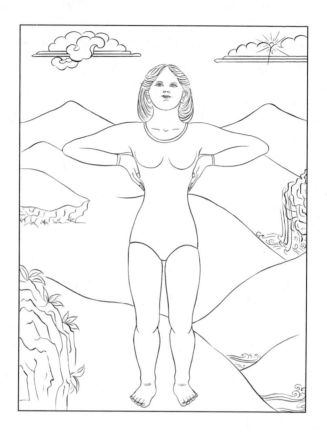

Exercise 60   Relieving Negativity

Stand well balanced with your feet a comfortable distance apart, your back straight, and your arms relaxed at your sides. Bend your elbows and place your hands flat against the sides of your body, as close under the armpits as possible, with the fingers pointing straight down. This may be rather difficult to do at first, and you may need some experiments to find the easiest way to do it. Do not press your sides too hard.

Breathing softly through both nose and mouth, bend your knees, and with your heels on the floor and your back straight, lower your body as if sitting down in a low chair. When you have lowered a certain distance, you may find that tension somewhere prevents you from going further, and your heels begin to lift from the floor. Stop and locate the tension. Then let it go, and continue to lower with your back straight until you find a specific point of balance and energy. You may need to move up and down a little until you find the right place. (If you have done Exercise 59, you have already found it.) Your thighs may begin to shake.

When you find the point of balance, look up and hold this position for thirty seconds to one minute. If you feel pain in the arms, go into the sensations of pain as fully as you can. Then straighten your legs, and in a continuing movement bend forward at the waist to about waist level, and hold briefly, keeping your breathing slow and gentle. Without changing the rest of the position, slowly bend your knees until you reach the special point of balance and energy, and when your legs begin to shake, hold for thirty seconds to one minute, breathing softly through nose and mouth. You may feel sensations of energy at the base of the spine as well as in the thighs.

Now straighten your legs, raise your torso, and let your hands slide down your sides until the arms hang relaxed at your sides. Stand or sit for several minutes, expanding the feelings generated by this exercise.

Do the exercise three times, resting after every repetition. To complete it, sit in the sitting posture for five to ten minutes, continuing to expand the feelings within and around your body.

As you do this exercise, you may feel some painful sensations at first. Customarily we think of pain as something to be avoided. Yet if you can concentrate on the sensations which are produced by this exercise (and by other exercises which involve holding a position for a period of time), you can go beyond the mental concept of 'pain' to a source of new and vital energy.

As you concentrate, let your breathing merge with your sensations and transform them into healing energy. If you wish, hold the position mentioned in the exercise for just a few seconds at first. When you have had more experience with tapping the energy held within tension, you will be able to hold this position for several minutes or more.

This exercise will energize the lower body and chest, relieving negative psychological patterns such as holding back, and building strength and confidence.

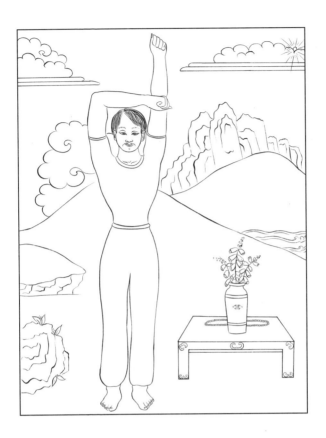

Exercise 61   Expanding Body Energy

Stand well balanced with your feet a few inches apart and
your arms relaxed at your sides. Make tight fists with both
hands. Extend your left arm in front of you at shoulder
height. Raise your right arm to shoulder height, bend it
at the elbow, and place the right fist under the left arm,
just above the elbow joint; the top of the fist (the thumb
and index finger) will touch the underside of the left arm.
Make sure the right elbow is at shoulder height.

Create strong opposing forces by pushing down with the left arm and up with the right. Maintain both strong tension and balance, and while inhaling through both nose and mouth, slowly raise both arms until the left arm is vertical and the right arm is bent over the head. The right arm should clear the head; if it does not, stretch the arms up slightly.

In this position, continuing to maintain the tension in the arms, exhale slowly, relaxing your belly, neck, and back. Then slowly lower your arms to shoulder height while inhaling, and as you do so, slowly release the tension in your arms. Let your breathing be smooth and easy throughout the movement. Lower your arms to your sides and rest for a minute, either standing or sitting, expanding the sensations produced by creating and releasing tension in this way.

Now reverse the position of the arms and repeat the movement, resting briefly afterward. Do the complete movement (once on each side) three times, resting after each side. At the end, sit in the sitting posture for five to ten minutes, continuing to expand the feelings stimulated by this movement.

This exercise, which can also be done sitting, relieves muscular tension, improves the circulation, and balances inner energies.

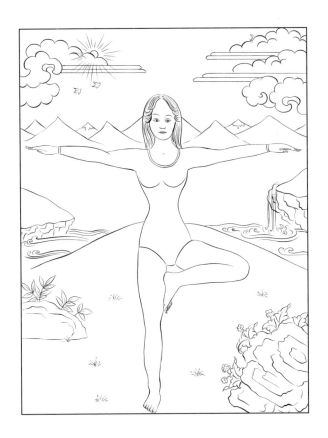

Exercise 62   Increasing Endurance

Stand barefoot and balance on your right leg with the sole of your left foot pressed against your upper right thigh, the heel resting near the crotch and the left knee out to the side. Lightly press the heel against the thigh to help keep the left foot in place. Without effort, slowly lift both your arms away from your sides, letting them float up until they are extended at slightly above shoulder height, with the palms down.

In this position, slowly turn at the waist to the right, and then to the left, keeping your head still and looking straight ahead with soft eyes. Move casually, breathing lightly and evenly, with your body loose and almost sleepy and your belly relaxed. Let the pressure of your left foot against your right thigh be as light as possible.

Then slowly lower your arms and leg at the same time, sensing the subtle changes in feeling as you come to balance again on both feet. Stand quietly for a minute. You may feel a release of tension in the neck and shoulders and a balanced feeling throughout your torso.

Now reverse the position of the legs, and repeat the movement. Do the complete movement, balancing first on one leg, then the other, three or nine times, standing briefly on both feet after each repetition. At the end, sit for five to ten minutes, expanding the feelings stimulated by the exercise.

This exercise balances body energy, and develops the ability to stay balanced during critical points of emotional or psychological change.

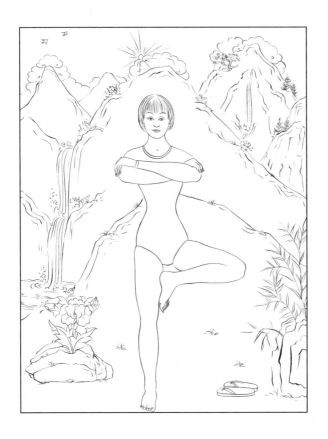

Exercise 63   Embracing Space

Stand barefoot and balance on your right leg with the sole
of your left foot pressed against your upper right thigh, and
your left knee out to the side. Slowly lift your arms in front
of you to shoulder height and then cross them, holding the
arms tightly just above the elbow. Bit by bit raise your arms
over and a little behind your head, stretching upward. Let
your neck settle down between the shoulders. Look toward
the ceiling, open your mouth, and stretch a little bit more.

Balance casually in this position. Loosen your belly; you may then find you can stretch a little more. Your upper back may be slightly arched.

Now slowly unfold your arms, with the palms toward the ceiling, until your arms straighten overhead. In a slow, uninterrupted motion, lower your arms to your sides, as if drawing angel wings in snow. Allow your hands and chest to open. When the arms reach your sides, lower the leg to the floor, until you are standing on both feet. Notice the special flavors of feeling that come just before your foot touches the floor.

Now reverse the position of your legs and repeat the movement. This time inhale as you stretch your tightly crossed arms upward. Hold the inhalation for a few seconds, with your arms overhead; then begin to exhale as you open your arms upward, and continue to exhale as your arms float down to your sides. The arm gesture can be generous and expressive, opening the chest and embracing space, extremely slow and gentle.

Do the complete movement (first one side and then the other) three times, coordinating your breathing with the movement. When you finish, stand silently on both feet for several minutes, your arms relaxed at your sides; then sit for five to ten minutes. You may feel a deep calm within your bones, especially the bones of your arms and chest.

This exercise may also be done standing on both feet, or else sitting.

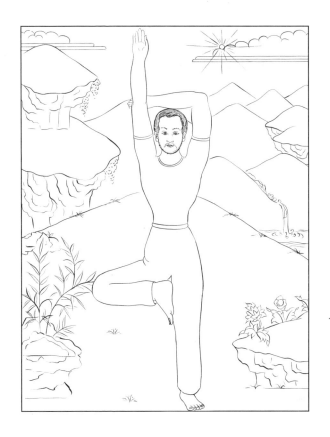

Exercise 64   Increasing Psychological Balance

Stand barefoot and balance on your left leg with the sole of your right foot against your upper left thigh and your right knee out to the side. Slowly extend your right arm in front of you at shoulder height, palm down. Place the left palm on top of the right elbow, with your left elbow at shoulder height. Push your right arm up toward the ceiling while strongly resisting this movement with your left arm. As you do this, relax the belly as much as you can, and breathe evenly and softly through both nose and mouth. When both arms are overhead, slowly release the tension and lower your arms to the first position, sensing the feelings that arise in and around your body.

Do the movement three times; then reverse the position of your legs and arms and do the exercise three times on the other side. At the end, sit in the sitting posture for five to ten minutes, following and expanding the feelings generated by this exercise.

This exercise is very calming to the nervous system. However, if you practice it when you are nervous or upset, you may need to begin the 'balancing process' by sitting quietly for ten or fifteen minutes, breathing gently and evenly through both nose and mouth. When you begin the exercise, move very slowly, bringing breath, awareness, and motion into a unity. The exercise will continue to calm and balance your mind and body.

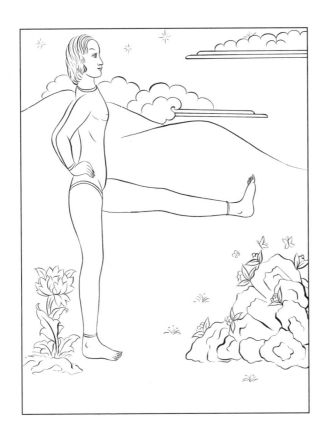

Exercise 65   Sameness of Inner and Outer

Stand barefoot on the floor, well balanced, with your back straight and your hands on your hips. Slowly bend your left knee and raise it toward your chest. Flex your left ankle so the toes point to the ceiling (the foot stays in this position throughout the movement). With your back straight and your belly relaxed, slowly straighten your left leg in front of you, with a slight kick at the very end of the stretch. At the same time, push your chest forward a little.

When straight, the leg is as nearly horizontal as possible. Then without putting the foot down, twice more draw your leg up toward your chest and slowly straighten it. The movement has the quality of slow leg stretches. After three leg stretches, very slowly, almost casually, lower your left leg to the floor. Notice any special flavors of feeling that come just before your foot meets the ground.

Now slowly lift your right knee and do the exercise on the other side. Without effort, maintain control of the movement throughout, keeping it smooth and slow. Watch the tension in your belly to gauge your level of anxiety. When you tighten your belly in order to exert control, you lose touch with precious energies which bring vitality. If you can be casual at critical points in the movement without forcing control, you will discover certain vital qualities and energies.

Do the complete movement, first on one side and then on the other, three times, and then sit for five to ten minutes, following and extending the feelings stimulated by this exercise. When you are familiar with the exercise, try it nine times, sitting for five to ten minutes after each set of three movements. This exercise improves coordination, increases body energy, and relieves tension in the chest.

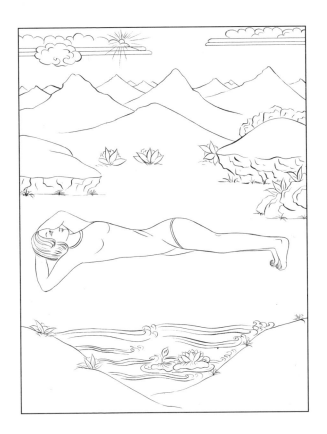

Exercise 66   Increasing Inner Balance

Lie on your right side with your legs straight, the left leg on top of the right. Interlace your fingers and place them behind your head so that your head rests on your right arm and your left elbow points to the ceiling. In this position, slowly begin to stretch, moving your left hip toward the floor in front of you, and at the same time, moving your left elbow to the left until you look up at the ceiling and your left shoulder comes near the floor.

Notice that as your hip moves forward, the legs may turn so that you can stand on your toes. Although it is possible to stretch until the lower half of the body faces the floor and the upper half faces the ceiling, do not be concerned if you do not stretch this far. Move easily, without straining; it does not matter how far you stretch.

Hold the stretch for thirty seconds to a minute, breathing softly through both nose and mouth. Gently increase the stretch as subtle tensions are released. Then slowly return to the original position, expanding the sensations awakened by this stretch.

Now roll onto your left side and repeat the stretch. Notice on which side of the body the stretch is easier. Do the complete exercise, to the right and left, three times. Then rest on your back (with your knees bent, if you wish) for five minutes, continuing to expand the sensations stimulated by the exercise.

This exercise gives inner balance to both the upper and lower body.

Stimulating and Transforming Energies

The body is like a vessel filled and surrounded by space.
The whole body exercises in space.

Energy is continuously being channeled through our bodies, from cell to cell, between mind and body, as well as between ourselves and the world around us. As we move and experience, even as we breathe, the energies within and around us continuously interact. We tend to think of energy and matter as opposites, but even the most solid objects are made up of moving energies: matter and energy are, on all levels, equivalent. Our physical bodies are much less solid than they seem. They are not fixed and impervious 'objects', but essentially flowing and open, participating in an ongoing process of 'embodiment' of energies.

When these energies flow smoothly, we have access to all the energy we could hope for. The body becomes healthy, and the mind clear. When this flow of energy is active and balanced, it regenerates every aspect of our bodies, minds, and senses, continuously increasing our mental and physical vitality. Feelings of love and openness nourish and renew us, radiating to the surrounding environment. All our experience participates in this rich, ongoing process of enjoyment and embodiment.

When we prevent this completely open flow, slowing the energies down and misdirecting them, our experience becomes contracted. We mentally freeze our sensations by concentrating on our thoughts about them. Instead of experiencing our sensations directly, letting them flow to our hearts where they deepen into nourishing joy and satisfaction, we judge. We become like bees, tapping beautiful flowers for pollen, but never enjoying the honey.

Looking for sensation and satisfaction, we direct our energies outwards. We fill the mind with ideas and expectations of what we want for the future, instead of enjoying what is at hand. We skim over the surface of our feelings. In order to 'feel more' we may direct our energy into our emotions, which quickly and easily feed us strong sensations. But these sensations are imbalanced, and cannot truly satisfy us —they stir up dissatisfaction instead of fulfillment. Psychological tensions then manifest on the physical level, automatically producing more tightening, which is reflected in negative patterns of thought, feeling, and action.

When our ability to contact our senses diminishes, so our vitality also decreases. In reaction we may try to 'save our energy' by relying on external forms of energy rather than our own, but this only continues to undermine both our vitality and our health. We then try to heal ourselves, taking our bodies to one place and our heads to another, not realizing that the remedy for both is in the naturally wholesome energies of our sensations and feelings, and in the integration of our bodies and minds.

Relaxation can heal both body and mind by awakening our inner resources, opening us to feelings which are much more than physical or even mental sensations. Our ordinary feelings and sensations are of several different kinds, some relating to our body awareness, others relating to our sensory or mental awareness. During relaxation, interactions are stimulated among body, senses, breath, and mind, bringing these different kinds of awareness and feeling into contact with each other.

As they expand and accumulate, the feelings and energies flow together and become integrated; once they are integrated, they naturally stimulate each other, developing further within themselves. Then every sense impression, breath, and movement increases and deepens enjoyment, and experience comes alive in the body. A deep feeling of fulfillment flows through every vein and organ, gathering richness until the boundaries within the body dissolve and the very outline of the body melts into surrounding space. Then living becomes enjoyment, and stimulation becomes relaxation. The texture of space nourishes us.

When we discover the intimacy of direct experience, we see that everything that arises, each feeling and sensation, is a center of experience. We do not do or accomplish anything, for there is no experiencer; there is only experience. This knowledge gives the possibility of

new interactions with 'negative' emotions such as confusion or resistance, for we see that they too are flexible
forms of vital energy and experience which can open into
positive directions.

As you practice the exercises in this section, go more
deeply into the feelings generated, bringing body, mind,
and senses together. Expand your sensations, letting them
become vital and strong. As 'breath' and subtle mental
and physical energies become integrated, these sensations
become deeper and more expansive than our ordinary
sensations. As these feelings are channeled through our
senses, all of our sensations and feelings become vibrant
and alive, much richer than before. Our whole body grows
saturated with this quality of joyful vitality and becomes
profoundly wholesome: a body of knowledge.

When you touch a negative emotion or a tight place
in your body or mind, let these sleeping energies awaken.
Mix them with your rich and joyful sensations, balance
your breath, and keep your awareness open, without
focusing too strongly. Stay with the feelings; let them
become exhilarating. Penetrate them with awareness and
breath. With enough concentration, you can actually
transform these feelings by a process of inner alchemy.

While practicing Kum Nye, you may experience energy centers opening. As the head center opens, it becomes
easy to think and communicate clearly. Visionary powers become possible. Intuitive powers develop when the

throat center opens, revealing to us the symbolic world of poetry and art. When the heart center opens, separation between ourselves and others dissolves, and we become a part of everything. Craving and grasping cease when the navel center opens, and a quality of energy like heat warms the whole body.

Once we learn to stimulate our feelings and energies through the practice of Kum Nye, we can expand them more and more each day, cultivating enjoyment and playfulness in every action. We can even enjoy stressful situations, because we can replenish our energy whenever we grow tired. Everything we do gives us more energy.

Directed like the point of a bright beam, each moment of life kindles accomplishment, enabling us to develop genuine perseverance and patience, without struggle or fixation. Then we can naturally do and simultaneously enjoy all the content of experience. We can fully appreciate the process of living within our 'body of knowledge' so that all mental and physical experience of living automatically continues to expand. Experience just opens of itself, naturally.

Without trying to possess them, we can let feelings of enjoyment stream through us and outside us, stimulating harmonious interactions in the world around us. Anything we contact, through sound, touch, or any of the senses, becomes radiant with subtle energy. Even walking or looking in a relaxed, open way allows the special light quality of universal energies to enter our bodies; then we can cultivate and expand that feeling until it permeates our bodies and spreads out from us into the universe. We participate in a continuous circle of living energies, a dance of appreciation, a commingling.

Stage One

Like the exercises in "Balancing and Integrating Body, Mind, and Senses," these exercises are divided into three stages in order of difficulty. Each stage is equivalent to the corresponding stage in the previous chapter. You may want to move back and forth between chapters in exploring the exercises at a given stage.

You may also want to explore some of the exercises in Stages Two and Three before completing all the exercises in the first stage. Let your body and your feelings guide you in selecting exercises to practice. However, if you find that you are racing through the exercises without going deeply into any of them, slow down and follow the progression of exercises given here. Remember to do each exercise completely, either three or nine times, and when it is appropriate, on both sides of the body.

Each exercise, no matter how simple on the surface, can unlock the treasure-house of experience in your body and mind. During the exercise, it is best not to be concerned with whether your feeling is good or bad—just feel it. Do not let the feelings mentioned in the exercise descriptions create expectations you feel you must meet in order to 'succeed' at the exercise. Simply tune your sensations, tune your breath, tune your awareness; then, although you may think 'nothing special' is happening, Kum Nye yoga will naturally vitalize even the most subtle layers of your body, mind, and senses. After practicing, observe the quality of your experience during the day. Even within a short time you will notice a more vibrant quality to daily life and your capacity for enjoyment will increase.

The exercises in this stage are simple to do. Practice them slowly, with sensitive attention to any sensations that occur throughout the whole body. Exercise 72, in particular, when practiced regularly over a period of at least one week, will greatly increase your awareness of the energy 'centers'. As these centers become more open, and internal organs and muscles are deeply massaged, a warm, gentle, satisfying feeling begins to nurture and sustain you. As this process deepens, these harmonious feelings nurture those around you as well.

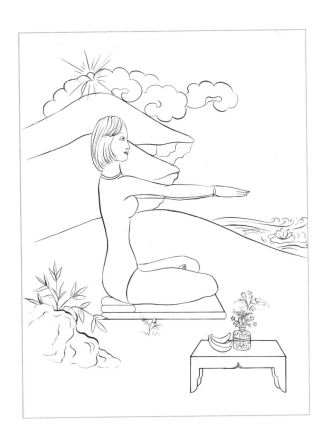

Exercise 67   Sensing Energy

Sit cross-legged on a mat or cushion and slowly extend
your arms in front of you at shoulder height, palms down.
Keeping your belly relaxed, move your hands backward by
pulling your shoulders back. Then reach forward with your
hands. Without hurrying, move your arms back and forth
in this way nine times. The rest of the body remains still.
Let the motion and the mind become inseparable. Then
find a place of balance in the shoulder sockets, neither

forward nor back, and lower your hands to your knees. Sit for three to five minutes, allowing the feelings and currents of energy stimulated by this movement to expand.

Once again extend your arms in front of you, and bend your arms at the elbow until the fingers are pointing toward the ceiling. Relax your neck as you do this movement. Then bit by bit lower your forearms until your arms are outstretched in front of you. Your upper arms remain still as your forearms move down very subtly. Feel the energy in your chest, within your heart center; there may be a feeling there of something moving down. Put your entire consciousness into whatever you feel; the feeling then becomes consciousness. Do this movement nine times, breathing softly and evenly through both nose and mouth; then lower your hands to your knees and sit for five to ten minutes.

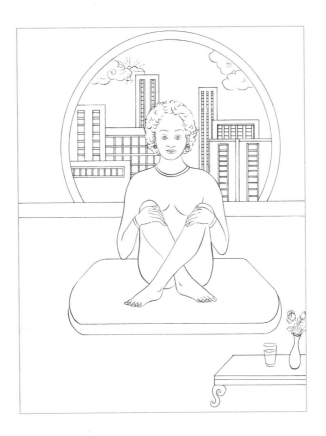

Exercise 68   Clearing Confusion

Sit on a rug or a flat mat and cross your legs in the manner
illustrated in the drawing. Take hold of your right ankle
with your right hand and your left ankle with your left
hand, and draw your feet along the floor as close to your
body as you can.

Place your hands just below the kneecaps and draw the
knees as close as possible toward your chest, keeping your
back straight and your shoulders down. If possible, touch

your knees to your chest. Look straight ahead and hold for one to three minutes, breathing softly through both nose and mouth, and concentrating lightly on your belly. (Count outbreaths to measure time if you wish.)

Now very slowly release the tension—take about one minute for this—feeling the sensations that arise in your body. Sit quietly in the sitting posture for a few minutes, continuing to explore these sensations. Then repeat the exercise, reversing the position of the legs as you cross them. Do the exercise three or nine times, sitting for a few minutes after each repetition, and for five to ten minutes at the end.

This exercise energizes the navel center and clears confusion from the mind.

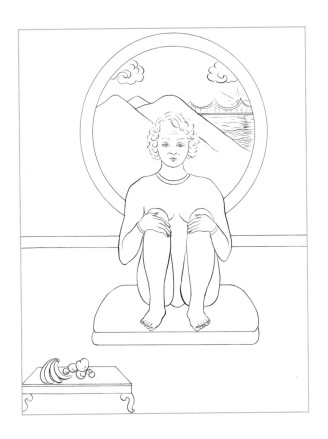

Exercise 69   Clear Mind

This exercise differs from the preceding exercise in the position of the legs. Sit on a rug or flat mat with your knees bent and your feet flat on the floor in front of you. Take hold of the left ankle with your left hand and the right ankle with your right hand. Draw your feet along the floor as close to your body as you can. Then place your hands just below the kneecaps and draw your knees as close to your chest as possible, keeping your back straight and your shoulders down. If possible, touch your knees to your chest. Look straight ahead and hold for one to three minutes, breathing softly through both nose and mouth, and concentrating lightly on your belly. (Count outbreaths to measure time if you wish.)

Now very slowly release the tension—take about one minute for this—going deeply into the sensations stimulated in your body. Sit quietly in the sitting posture for a few minutes, continuing to expand these sensations. Repeat the exercise three or nine times, sitting for several minutes after each repetition, and for five to ten minutes at the end.

This exercise, like the preceding one, increases energy in the lower energy center and brings clarity to the mind.

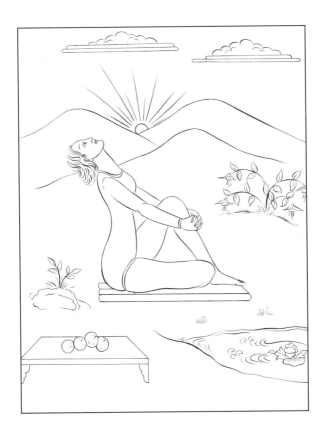

Exercise 70   Light Energy

Do this exercise very gently if you are pregnant or have
had any neck or back injuries, or if you have had an operation within the last three or four months.

Sit on the floor (not on a mat or cushion) with your
legs loosely crossed, the left leg outside of the right. Raise
your left knee and bring your left heel in front of your right
ankle, with the sole of your left foot on the floor. Interlace
your fingers and clasp your left knee with your hands.

Gradually arch the spine and neck backwards. Do not let your head go all the way back; the curve in the spine is graceful and not extreme. To strengthen the arch, gently pull on your knee. Keep your right knee on the floor if you can. Do not stretch too strenuously. Hold the stretch for three to five minutes, breathing gently and evenly through both nose and mouth. Concentrate lightly on energy moving up your spine.

When you feel heat at the back of your neck, take time to release the tension. You may take at least a minute to straighten the spine, expanding feelings of warmth and energy. Do this exercise three times on one side.

Then reverse the position of the legs and do the exercise three times on the other side. Sit quietly for ten minutes at the conclusion of the exercise, allowing the feelings stimulated by the movement to radiate like a halo. This exercise releases tension in the spine.

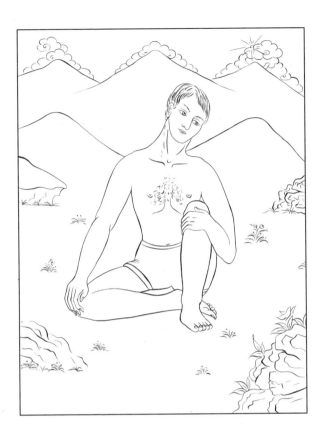

Exercise 71   Releasing Tension

Sit on a mat or cushion with your legs loosely crossed, the
left leg outside the right. Raise your left knee and bring
your left heel in front of your right ankle, with the sole of
your left foot flat on the floor or mat. Draw your feet as
close to your body as you can, and place your hands on
your knees.

Now slowly and gently stretch your neck back and to
the left, so that your right arm straightens and your head

and neck come into a line with your right arm. Keep the right knee down. Hold the diagonal stretch for about thirty seconds, breathing gently and evenly through both nose and mouth.

Release the tension gradually, taking thirty seconds to one minute to do so. Let your breath and awareness flow with the sensations awakened in your body. Sit quietly for a few minutes, allowing sensations to flow and expand. Reverse the position of your legs and stretch the neck toward the other side. Rest briefly afterward.

Do the complete exercise, first on one side, then the other, three or nine times, resting for a few minutes after each side. Be sure to release the tension very slowly. At the end of the exercise, sit in the sitting posture for five to ten minutes, continuing to expand the sensations generated by the stretch.

This exercise releases tension in the neck, shoulders, and head; it can relieve headache.

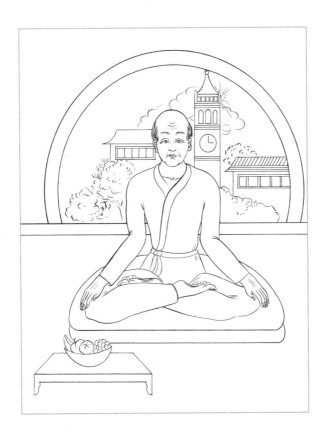

Exercise 72   Embodiment

Sit comfortably in the sitting posture. Concentrate on
the energy center below the navel for half an hour a day
for three days. Breathe gently and evenly through both
nose and mouth, and keep your eyes half-open if possible. Sometimes it is easier in the beginning to close the
eyes, and this is also all right. Begin by doing whatever
you do when you concentrate. After two days, change the
quality of the concentration so it becomes less forceful,

and there is simply a quality of awareness. With this kind of concentration, your body energy will flow: calm feelings arise gradually, and thoughts slow down.

At times the feeling is soft and gentle, like warm milk, very thick, rich, and deep. Become very still and expand the feelings; this will make them last longer. Feel them as much as you can, and send them to all the different parts of your body—up to your face and neck, and down to your feet and toes. Subtly hold the breath, just a little tightly, in the lower part of the belly and in the sacrum; then expand the feelings to your whole body, more and more, until it is as if the whole universe were to become those feelings. The feelings blow like a warm summer breeze in a hot place, healing you within and without, passing through many layers of your body: first your skin, in and between the surface tissues and nerves; then deeper within, to nerves, tissues, and organs. Sometimes the feelings move deep within like a little whirl of wind.

After you have concentrated on the navel center in this way for half an hour a day for three days, move to the heart center and concentrate there for an equal amount of time. Then move to the throat center, and finally, to the head center, between the eyes.

If you would like to try concentrating in this way for a longer period of time, concentrate on each energy center for half an hour each day, for two or three weeks. Then certain experiences may occur. Colors—perhaps green or white light, or red, orange, blue, or mixed colors—may appear. You may see different objects, or feel various feeling-tones, or hear a high-pitched sound. If these or other experiences occur, do not become attached or fascinated by them. Simply allow them to happen, and expand the sensations as much as you can.

If too many thoughts make it difficult for you to sleep, lightly concentrate on the heart center for half an hour every evening for two weeks. Try not to think about anything; do not read or write after the exercise. Just go into the feeling in your heart center, deepening and expanding it until a joyful quality develops. Continue it, more and more, as if there were nothing else in the world, only this feeling.

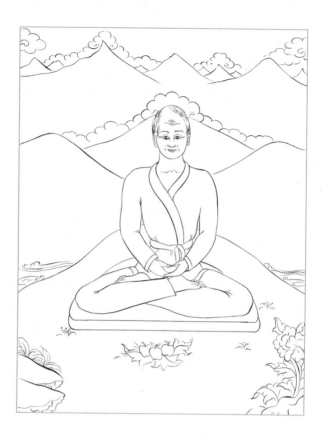

Exercise 73   Om Ah Hum

Sit in the sitting posture on a mat or cushion. Breathe softly through both nose and mouth. Think of the mantra Om Ah Hum, feeling Om in the head center at the top of the head, Ah in the throat center, and Hum in the heart center. Begin to chant the mantra inwardly, quite slowly.

Now silently chant Om with your hands on your knees. Then slowly move your hands in front of your belly with the palms up, and cradle the fingers of the right hand in the fingers of the left hand. Lift the thumbs a little and join them, as in the drawing. In this position, inwardly chant AH. Then slowly move your hands, palms up, to your knees, and rest them there, silently chanting HUM. Begin a new cycle by turning your hands over on your knees while chanting OM.

Continue in this way for twenty-five complete cycles, combining your inward chanting of the mantra with the movement. Let breath, chant, and movement become one. When you finish, sit quietly in the sitting posture for five to ten minutes, expanding the sensations awakened by this exercise. Throughout the day, silently remember OM AH HUM from time to time.

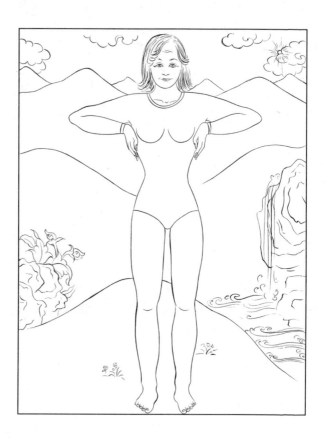

Exercise 74 Wholesome Vitality

Stand well balanced with your back straight, your arms relaxed at your sides, and your feet a comfortable distance apart, with the toes turned out slightly. Bend your elbows and place your hands flat against the sides of the body, as close under the armpits as possible, with the fingers pointing straight down. This may be a little hard to do at first. Do not press your sides too hard. Inhale deeply through both nose and mouth, then gently and silently hold the breath, and concentrate lightly on your chest. Relax your belly and tighten the buttocks a little. Then while still holding the breath, bend your knees slightly and hold. If you feel pain in your arms, go into the painful sensations as deeply as you can.

Now slowly exhale, and at the same time straighten your legs and glide your hands down the sides of the body until your arms hang relaxed at your sides. Let the contact between hands and body be as full as possible as you do this. Stand or sit for a few minutes, breathing gently through both nose and mouth, expanding the sensations in your body. You may feel heat in your chest and the back of your neck.

Do the exercise three times, standing or sitting briefly after each repetition. At the end, sit in the sitting posture for five to ten minutes, continuing to expand the feelings produced by the exercise. Your head may feel clearer, your heart more open, and your senses more alive.

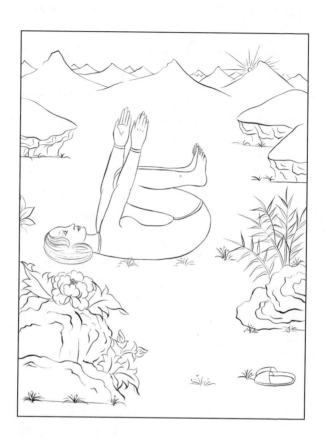

Exercise 75   Body of Energy

Lie on your back with the arms at your sides and the legs separated about the width of your pelvis. Bend your knees, one at a time, and place your feet flat on the floor. With the palms facing each other, slowly lift your arms to the ceiling. In this position, roll the pelvis and knees toward your chest, lifting them as high off the floor as possible. The back of your waistline will come off the floor, and your arms will move apart a little. Keeping your arms up, slowly roll back until your pelvis and feet rest on the floor. Breathe easily through both nose and mouth throughout the movement. Continue three times, expanding the sensations awakened by the roll.

Now do the movement quickly, six to nine times, breathing gently through both nose and mouth. Then straighten your legs one at a time, lower your arms to your sides and rest on your back for a few minutes, continuing to amplify and extend the feelings in and around your body.

Do the exercise three times (beginning with three slow rolls, then six to nine quick rolls), resting on your back after each repetition and at the end of the whole series.

This exercise releases tension that has built up in the muscles of the lower abdomen, relieving emotions, and refreshing the whole body.

Stage Two

The following exercises activate energies in specific areas of the body, including the hands, wrists, arms, chest, shoulders, back, thighs, legs, and toes. As you do them, distribute the sensations awakened in a particular place until your whole body participates in the 'massage'. You will find that the exercises which lengthen the muscles along the spine release particularly joyful sensations.

When an exercise involves a stretch, slowly ease into the stretch, breathing softly and evenly, developing a quality of lightness. Be sure not to stretch too much. Remember to 'hold' a position lightly too, breathing gently and releasing subtle tensions throughout your body. If you wish, use your breath to measure time by counting out breaths. Release holding or tension slowly, maintaining the quality of lightness, and allowing your sensations to expand.

When you notice a tight place in your body and mind, explore it, without dwelling on it. If you wish, use the tension as 'food' for Exercises 87 and 89. With continuing practice of Kum Nye yoga, tension will gradually melt, stimulating energy to flow evenly throughout your body until it cycles and recycles, constantly replenishing itself.

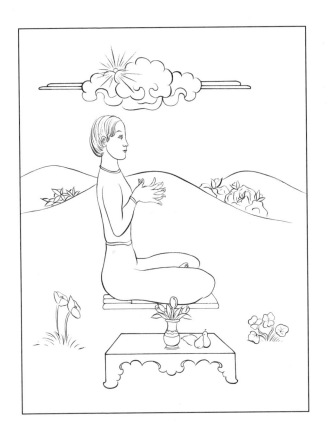

Exercise 76   Building Strength and Confidence

Sit cross-legged on a mat or cushion and press your palms
together with the fingers pointing straight ahead; then
press the heels of your hands into the center of your chest.
Keeping your palms pressed tightly together, separate
your fingers and thumbs from each other, and slowly and
steadily move them apart and back as much as possible,
with your elbows out and your shoulders down. Be sure
to press the palms together as you do this, and relax your

belly. The back of your neck will be a little stiff. Breathing softly through both nose and mouth, hold this position for three minutes, until your palms become heated. Then release the tension, feeling the sensations that arise.

Now do the exercise again, holding the position this time for five minutes, separating your fingers and thumbs as much as possible. After five minutes, release the tension slowly and bring your hands to your eyes, cupping them over your open eyes so that no light shines through. (Do not actually touch your eyes.) Look softly, opening to the inside of the energy. Can you feel something? There may be a sensation of warmth or flowing energy.

Now stare strongly into the dark cave made by your hands, breathing softly and evenly through both nose and mouth. Once you have heated up the palms, you can stare for as long as ten minutes. You may see tiny stars, vibrations, colors, light or darkness, or have very pleasurable feelings. After five to ten minutes, slowly lower your hands to your knees, and look around you slowly and gently. What do you feel? Is there a special quality or sensation to your seeing?

You can also bring your palms, once they are heated, to many other parts of your body. Try the following two suggestions, and then experiment on your own.

• Heat up your palms again, holding for five minutes, then put one hand crosswise on your chest and the other

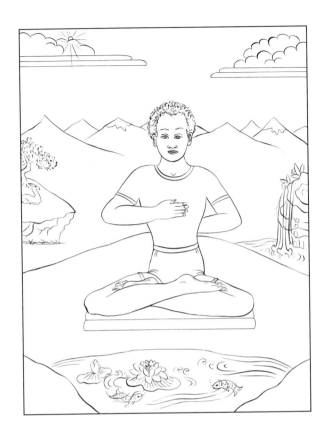

crosswise on the middle of your back. Let the whole hand come in contact with your body. Feel the warmth penetrate your chest and spine, as if you had no skin. After a few minutes, bring one hand to your forehead and the other to the back of your head and continue to sense the feelings expand in your body.

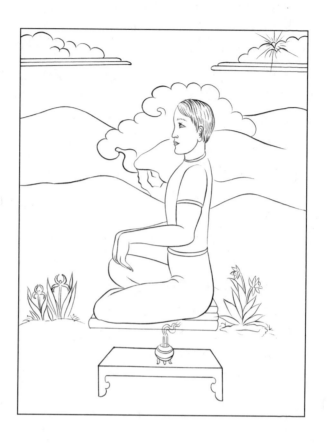

Exercise 77   Stream of Energy

Sit cross-legged on a mat or cushion with your back
straight. Lightly press your elbows to your sides, and lift
your forearms in front of you until they are roughly parallel to the floor, with the palms down. Breathing evenly
through both nose and mouth, lift your shoulders slightly
and hold, with your chest relaxed. Keeping the fingers and
thumb of each hand together, slowly bend your wrists so
your fingers point toward the floor. There is an arching

quality to this bending. Hold the hands down for a minute, with the rest of the body still and relaxed. Then very slowly lift your hands, releasing the tension and sensing the feelings stimulated in your hands, arms, chest, and the back of your neck. You may feel energy flowing through your wrists and arms to your heart center and spine. Allow whatever sensations you feel to expand.

Lower your hands to your knees and rest briefly. Then repeat the movement, this time increasing the bend in the wrist so your hands come closer to the underside of your forearm. Hold for one to five minutes before slowly releasing the tension. Do the movement three or nine times, resting briefly after each repetition. At the end, sit for five to ten minutes, expanding and distributing your sensations throughout your body, and beyond to the surrounding universe.

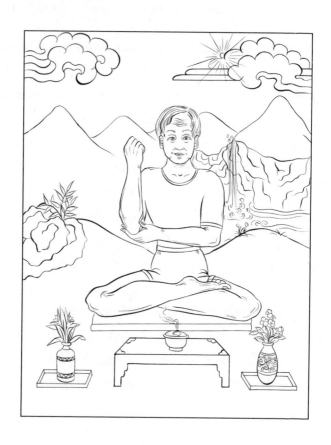

Exercise 78   Stimulating Body Energy

Sit cross-legged on a mat or cushion and bend your right
arm at the elbow so your right hand points to the ceiling with the palm facing you. Make a fist. Place your left
thumb and middle finger exactly on the ends or 'corners'
of the elbow crease (pressure points 5 and 6 in Figure 5,
page 125, Part One). Support your elbow from below with
your left palm and grasp it tightly, pressing strongly with
both thumb and middle finger. You may feel sensations

at the joint. Lift the elbow up a little so your right hand is at about the same height as your head.

Now, facing forward, slowly turn the torso and arms to the right, continuing to press strongly and steadily with your thumb and middle finger. Take about thirty seconds for this movement. Be sure to relax your neck (while still facing forward). Breathe very lightly through both nose and mouth, and let the breath bring more energy into your awareness.

When you have twisted to the right as far as you can comfortably go, return to the front, again taking about thirty seconds. Notice the quality of the movement in this direction. Then release the pressure of your thumb and middle finger, allowing your sensations to expand, and lower your hands to your knees. Sit for a few minutes, continuing to amplify the sensations in your body. You may feel stimulated in the chest or heart center.

Now reverse the position of the arms and repeat the movement to the left side, resting briefly afterward. Do the complete exercise, first one side, then the other, three or nine times, resting a minute after each repetition and for five to ten minutes at the end.

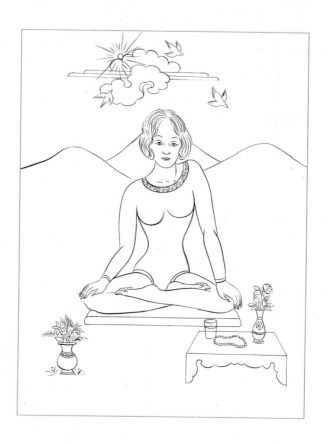

Exercise 79   Healing Energy

Sit cross-legged on a mat or cushion with your hands on your knees. Slowly raise your left shoulder as high as possible, and slowly lower your right shoulder as much as possible. As you raise the left shoulder, straighten your left arm, steadily pressing your hand against your leg. Move your right elbow slightly out to the side, so your right shoulder can lower more. Face straight ahead and let your head settle down between the shoulders.

Your left shoulder may come close to or even touch your left ear; do not, however, lean your head toward the shoulder. When you think you have stretched your shoulders apart as much as you can, relax for a few seconds. Then slowly stretch them apart a little more. Relax your lower belly and allow it to curve in a natural way. Hold the position for three to five minutes or more, breathing through nose and mouth, with your throat relaxed. It is important to be relaxed throughout this entire exercise.

Now gradually, in very slow motion, return your shoulders to their normal position. Take at least one minute to do this. Move as slowly as you can ever remember moving, and be aware of the interconnections among your feelings, senses, and awareness. You may feel a delicious warmth in your back and the back of your neck.

Now reverse the position of your shoulders and repeat the exercise. Do the complete exercise (first one side, then the other) three times. At the end, sit quietly for five to ten minutes, expanding and deepening your feelings and sensations. This exercise stimulates energy in the shoulders, neck, head, chest, and back.

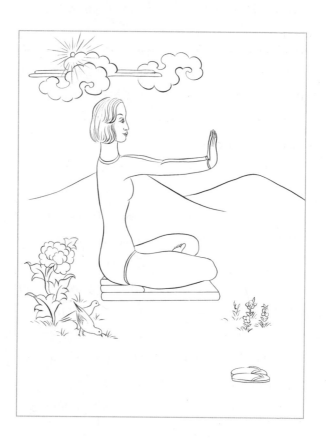

Exercise 80   Nurturing Satisfaction

Sit cross-legged on a mat or cushion with your hands
on your knees. Bend your arms at the elbow, lifting your
hands until they are in front of your shoulders with the
palms facing forward. Imagine that a great force is pushing against your hands, and slowly push it away. Let strong
tension build in your hands and arms, but relax your belly
and lower back, and breathe easily and lightly through
both nose and mouth. Keep pushing this force away

until your arms are stretched out in front of you. Your hands and arms may shake with tension. Then without releasing the tension—as if the force is more powerful than you—slowly move your arms back in front of your chest, keeping your belly relaxed.

Now very slowly release the tension—take about one minute for this—feeling the sensations in your arms, chest, and body. Notice the qualities of different stages of relaxation. Then slowly lower your hands to your knees and rest for a moment, continuing to expand the feelings that have been stimulated by producing and releasing tension in this way.

Do the exercise three times, resting briefly after each repetition. Then sit quietly in the sitting posture for five to ten minutes, continuing to expand the sensations in your body. You may feel an opening in your chest and upper back, and your breathing may become more open and free-flowing.

This exercise increases muscle strength in the arms and relieves tension throughout the upper body. It can also be done standing.

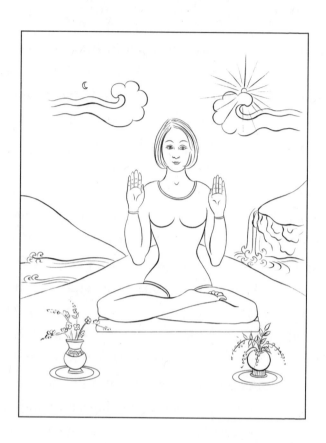

Exercise 81   Stimulating the Present Body

Sit cross-legged on a mat or cushion with your elbows held close against the sides of your body, your forearms vertical, and your palms facing forward. Imagine that you are pushing against the hands of someone stronger than you who is forcing the hands, arms, and shoulders back. Very slowly move your arms and shoulders back, letting the tension build. Your fingers may tremble. Take at least one minute for this movement. Let the spine, neck, and chest be straight and very still; this will help to increase the energy. Relax your belly and lower back.

Now release the tension over a period of a minute, letting the arms move forward in the same plane. As you do this, look inward into the heart. Let your awareness be so sensitive that you can feel the subtle changes that occur in each instant. You may experience a deep emotional feeling like relief or real satisfaction. Perhaps there is a sensation of deep relaxation around your heart, and a melted quality to all of your muscles. You may feel sensations of heat or cold in the spine.

Slowly lower your hands to your knees and rest a minute, continuing to expand your sensations. Repeat the exercise three times, resting briefly after each repetition. At the end sit for five minutes or more, feeling the silent quality of this relaxation. As you continue to practice this exercise, hold your arms back for longer periods of time and slow down the process of release even more.

Like the preceding exercise, this exercise builds muscle strength in the arms and relieves tension in the upper body.

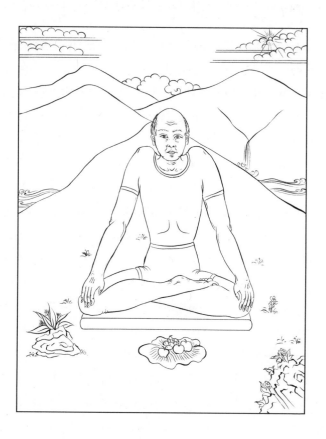

Exercise 82   Inner Massage

Sit cross-legged on a mat or cushion with the hands on your knees. With your lower body as relaxed as possible, move your shoulder blades back toward each other, squeezing the big muscles along the sides of the spine. In this position, slowly raise your shoulders as high as you can, settling your neck down between them in such a way that you are almost pushing your neck down, and your chin comes close your chest. Feel the backbone lifting all the way down to your sacrum. With your shoulder blades in the same position, slowly lower your shoulders, massaging down the spinal muscles. Now slowly, expanding your feelings, release the tension.

Do the exercise again, this time coordinating your breathing with the movement. Inhale as you raise your shoulders; then briefly hold the breath in your chest, with your stomach a little held in. Slowly lower your shoulders, and begin to exhale when your shoulders are at a nearly normal level. Exhale so slowly and smoothly that the exhalation becomes almost silent. Continue the exercise, three or nine times, then sit quietly for five to ten minutes.

• Now try this variation. Move your shoulder blades back toward each other and slowly raise your shoulders as high as possible, simultaneously pushing your neck down into your body with your chin close to your chest. Then very slowly relax the tension, lifting your head as if someone were pulling you up from the top of your head, and at the same time letting the shoulders move down. Concentrate on the upward movement of the head and feel the upward stretch along the length of your backbone. You may feel sensations of lightness and energy throughout a central column in your body, and a healing feeling in the center of the bones, a special kind of energy and warmth.

Repeat the spinal massage three times. Then sit for five to ten minutes, exercising the sensations and feelings.

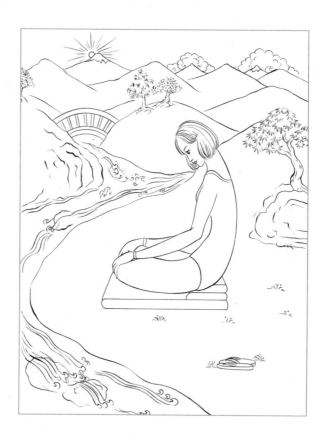

Exercise 83   Stimulating Vital Energy

Sit cross-legged on a mat or cushion with your hands resting on your knees. Visualize the spine as a slightly arching bow, without actually bending forward. Flatten your belly against your spine and lightly push out the spine of the middle back, as if pushing the vertebrae apart. The movement in your spine can be quite subtle. As you do this, relax your hands and lower your head a little, while keeping your chest up. Hold this position for three to five minutes, breathing gently and evenly through both nose and mouth, and concentrating lightly on lengthening the spine of your middle back.

After three to five minutes, slowly straighten your spine, feeling warm, calm, healing energy flow through the whole length of your spine, relaxing you and bringing a sensitive, joyful sensation. Sit quietly for a minute, continuing to expand the sensations in your body.

Do the exercise three or nine times, sitting briefly each repetition. At the end, sit for five to ten minutes, expanding the sensations flowing through your spine to the rest of your body and beyond it to surrounding environment.

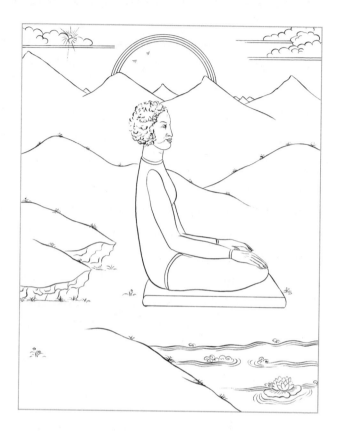

Exercise 84   Stimulating the Essence of Vitality

Sit cross-legged on a mat or cushion with your hands on your knees and your back straight. Breathe easily through both nose and mouth. Slowly begin to compress the spine, letting each vertebra sink down close to the next, all the way down your spine, until you feel the root of your body sink into the ground. Take at least a minute to do this, continuing to breathe slowly and evenly through both nose and mouth. Go deeply into the sensations of this movement.

Now, beginning at the base of your spine, begin to lift the vertebrae away from each other, feeling space open within as well as between the bones. Do this slowly, letting the spaces expand and flow together until they have no boundaries. Let the subtle energy of the breath enter and become part of this vast, expanding space.

When you lift the spine of your neck, imagine that the top of your head is being drawn toward the sky. Feel the sensation of space expanding as you stretch upwards. Taste the special quality of this relaxation. Sit for three to five minutes, expanding your sensations. Do the exercise three times, sitting for a few minutes after each repetition and for five to ten minutes at the end.

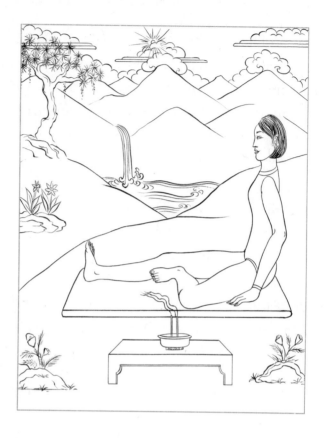

Exercise 85   Being and Energy

Sit on the floor or ground with your palms on the floor near your hips and your right leg stretched out in front of you. Flex your right ankle so the toes point toward your head and place your left foot against the inside of your right knee, with your left knee on the floor, if possible.

Now push your left foot against your right knee, and push your right knee against your left foot until your legs are almost shaking. You may be able to push harder with

338

the left leg than with the right. Hold the tension for thirty seconds to one minute, with your belly relaxed, breathing easily through both nose and mouth. Then release the tension and remain in this position, expanding the sensations in your body.

Now reverse the position of the legs and repeat the exercise. Do the complete movement, first one side, then the other, three times. When you finish, sit in the sitting posture for five to ten minutes, continuing to expand your feelings and sensations.

This exercise activates pressure points on the knee and foot. (See Figures 7 and 8, on pp. 135 and 141 respectively) Especially as you release the pressure, unify breath, awareness, and sensation, allowing the many subtle flavors of feeling to merge and expand.

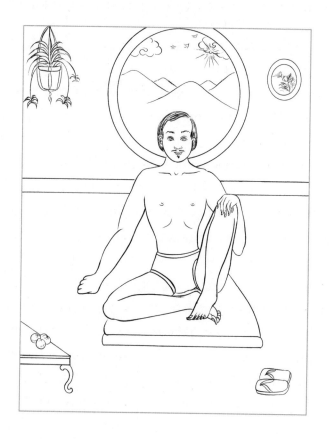

Exercise 86   Stimulating Healthy Feeling

Sit barefoot on the floor or ground with your legs loosely crossed, the right leg outside the left.

Make a fist with your left hand, and turn the fist so the inner side of it—the index finger and the thumb—is pointing toward the floor. Place the fist in this position on the floor quite close behind you, so you are supported by your left arm. Lift the right knee and place the right foot across the left foot, arch to arch, with the toes and the ball of the right foot on the floor. Place the right hand on your right knee.

Now slowly rock forward and backward: push your right knee down toward the floor, lift your left hip, standing on your right toes, and at the same time stretching your upper body backward a little. Be careful not to stretch your toes too much. Then, without holding, rock back onto your pelvis. Notice that as you do this movement, the arches of both feet are massaged. If you find the exercise difficult to perform with the left hand in a fist, try it with the palm flat on the floor. Also try placing the left hand at different distances from your body; the stretch will be stronger when the hand is nearer the body.

Stretch the toes in this way three or nine times on the right side, then reverse the position of your arms and legs and repeat the movement three or nine times on the left side. Then sit in the sitting posture for five to ten minutes, expanding the sensations produced by releasing tension and stimulating pressure points in this way.

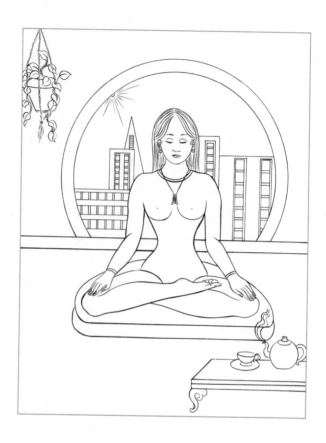

Exercise 87   Transmuting Negative Energies

Sit cross-legged on a mat or cushion with your hands on your knees and close your eyes in a relaxed way. Softly and gently feel warmth and a kind of sweetness in a place where you feel tight and uncomfortable. Subtle, accepting feelings will come. At first focus there; then apply less and less concentration, while still experiencing the subtle qualities of feeling. Listen to the feelings with your internal senses. Attend to how the feeling enters your heart, throat, back, the back of your neck, your lower stomach, your hands, your skin—wherever you have sensation of holding or tightness. Let every cell in your body be relaxed; hold nothing. Let tension in your forehead go, and relax the areas around the eyes and ears.

Let subtle energies float and find new pathways in your body. Let the looseness of your concentration become a feeling quality, as if you were lightly swimming or swaying. In a light way, keep increasing the sensation of movement. Expand the feeling, going deeper and deeper, beyond what seem to be the limits of the feeling. Let the feeling become larger until finally there is nothing but the feeling, and your mind and senses become one. Thoughts, concepts, and feelings merge together, mind and senses flow together, embracing each other, merging totally.

At first concentrate like this for twenty minutes at a time, once or twice a day for a week. If you would like to explore further, continue your internal listening and expansion of these subtle feelings for an hour each day for a month.

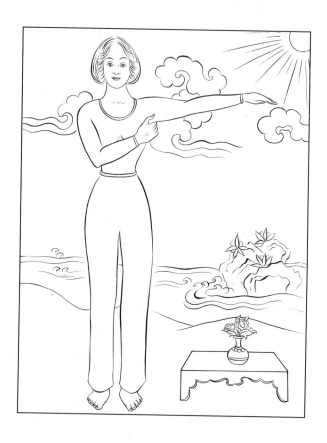

Exercise 88   Stimulating Inner Body Energies

Stand well balanced with your back and neck straight and your feet a comfortable distance apart. Slowly stretch out your right arm to the side at shoulder height, with the palm down. With your left hand, grasp the muscle which connects the right shoulder and arm, putting your fingers in the armpit and pressing with your thumb a pressure point on the right extremity of the chest. (This is point 7 in Figure 5, page 125, Part One.)

Hold the muscle firmly and push it upward and into your chest. Keeping your arm straight and your palm down, slowly rotate your right arm in the largest circle possible. Breathe gently through both nose and mouth and look straight ahead, with your back straight and your head still. Very slowly, taking about one minute for each circle, draw three or nine circles; then find a place where it feels natural to change direction and draw three or nine circles the other way. When you finish, stand without moving for a few minutes, with your eyes closed, and feel the flow of energies in your body. Be aware of sensations in your chest, especially the heart and lung areas.

Now repeat the slow circles with your left arm, three or nine times in each direction. Try making some of the circles different sizes to produce different tones of feeling. Then sit for five to ten minutes, expanding the sensations quickened by this exercise.

• Here is another version of the above exercise. Raise your right arm overhead and make a fist. With the left hand, grasp the muscle on the right side of the chest in the manner described above. Hold the muscle firmly and push it upward and into your chest. Keeping your arm straight, very slowly rotate your right arm forward, drawing the largest circle possible to the side of your body. Your arm will move close to your right leg and near your right ear during the slow rotation. Breathe very easily and relax your belly and spine; only the arms are slightly tensed. Make three or nine slow circles in this direction, then three or nine slow circles in the opposite direction. Pay close attention to feelings in your shoulders, back, neck, and chest.

When you have completed the circles with your right arm, stand quietly for a few minutes to feel the sensations in your body. Then very slowly repeat the movement with your left arm. Make sure that the circles are at the side of your body, and remember to breathe gently and evenly through both nose and mouth. At the conclusion of the exercise, sit in the sitting posture for five to ten minutes, feeling the movement of energies within you.

Like Exercise 94 and other exercises and massages, this exercise combines movement with pressure on a certain point. You might want to try pressing the point before beginning the movement, going deeply into the feelings that are produced. Then develop the movement, using it to deepen, distribute and expand your sensations. Experiment with various degrees of pressure as the arm rotates, following the changes in feeling-tone during each part of the movement. Be sure to release the pressure on the point slowly and gradually.

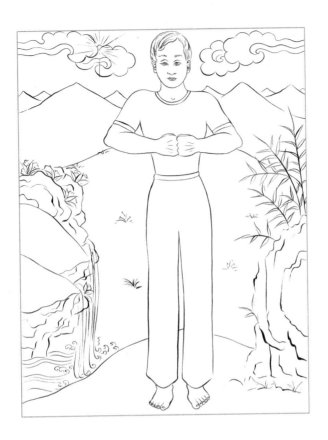

Exercise 89   Transforming Energy

Stand well balanced with your feet a comfortable distance apart, your back straight, and your arms at sides. Clench your fists strongly, hold your breath back in the chest, and tighten your chest until you feel something similar in quality to anger.

Then breathing lightly—without losing the intense feeling of holding back in the chest—bring the elbows and fists up until they reach chest height. Strongly press your fists together knuckle to knuckle, and place them in the center of your chest.

Make your body and fists strong and tense. Inhale deeply so the breath rolls down into the belly and draws energy from the base of the spine up into your chest. Hold this energy back internally with the breath and with your chest, as if protecting yourself. Intensify the feeling of blocking and holding back as much as you can, so your energy becomes concentrated.

Now with your body still, suddenly thrust your arms straight out, palms forward, releasing the gathered energy in an explosion. While fully and sharply exhaling, shout HA from your chest. It is important for this arm movement to be straight forward, and for the hands to be bent up at the wrists. Every aspect of the tension— physical, mental and emotional—is released simultaneously. Stay for a moment in this position with outstretched arms, fingers wide. In the pause after the explosion, what is the feeling?

Lower the arms to your sides and stand quietly for a few minutes. Do the exercise three times, standing briefly after each repetition. Then sit in the sitting posture for five to ten minutes, expanding the sensations stimulated by producing and releasing tension in this way. It is possible to do this exercise nine times, repeating the pattern of alternating exercise and sitting three times.

Through this exercise, mental agitation and emotional discomfort can be transformed. As soon as the energy is disconnected from a particular pattern, a totally new way of being can form. Try this when you feel tired, depressed, negative, or blocked. The exercise can be done sitting.

Once you are entirely familiar with this exercise, try the following variations:

• Do the exercise as described above. After releasing the tension and shouting HA, stay for a moment with outstretched arms, expanding the feeling at the pause. As you lower your arms, gather that feeling and bring it into your body. Stand quietly for a few minutes; then repeat the exercise twice more. Sit afterward for five to ten minutes, continuing to exercise your sensations: expanding them, then drawing them back into your body.

• This variation develops a subtle inner transformation. Do the exercise as described in the first version. After releasing the tension and shouting HA, remain in the pause for a moment. As you slowly let your arms down, gently hold the breath up in your chest until it dissolves into a subtle inner feeling or 'breath' in the chest. When it becomes too hard to hold the breath in, let it gradually ease down to a point of balance lower in your body. When it becomes too difficult to hold the breath at this point, let it move down to a lower point of balance. Continue this process, gradually lowering the breath in your body until the sensation can hardly be felt. Then repeat the exercise.

Do the exercise three times. Then sit quietly for ten to fifteen minutes, allowing this subtle inner feeling of breath to expand.

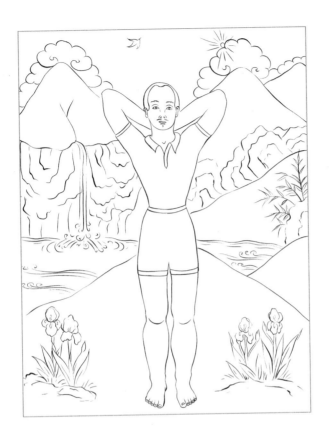

Exercise 90   Living Breath

Stand well balanced with your feet a comfortable distance apart, your back straight, and your arms relaxed at your sides. Interlace your fingers and place them at the back of your neck, with the elbows wide apart and your chest high. Breathe gently through both nose and mouth.

Bend your knees a little and arch your spine and neck slightly backwards. Make sure your chest is high and your body relaxed and balanced.

Then take two, three, or four quick, gasp-like intakes of breath from the belly, and exhale as slowly as possible, attending particularly to the sensations in your belly area. Let the breath massage you internally. Picture the breath passing from the bloodstream into all the internal organs, suffusing each cell, even each molecule, with vital, relaxing sensation. Try to sense the subtle inner quality of this massage of the breath.

Do the exercise three or nine times; then sit for five to ten minutes, continuing to expand the sensations of this internal massage. This exercise relieves tension in the belly area and lightens negative patterns such as resistance.

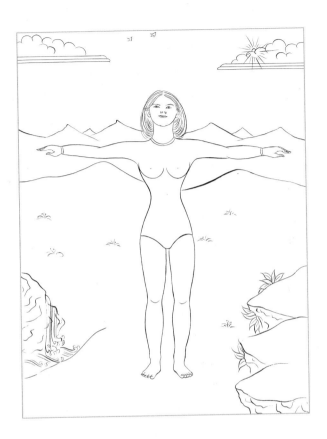

Exercise 91   Activating Healing Energy

Stand well balanced with your feet a few inches apart, your back straight, and your arms relaxed at your sides.

Stretch your arms out to your sides at shoulder height, with the palms facing down. Move your head backward a little bit so you look up at the point where the wall meets the ceiling. Relax your neck, open your mouth, and flare your nostrils. The breath flows in and out easily through both nose and mouth.

Now relax your belly and chest as fully as you can; bring your attention to the base of your spine, and tighten your buttocks. Hold for three to five minutes, continuously concentrating on the base of your spine. Be sure to keep your belly and chest very relaxed. If mild shaking or trembling develops, go into it and release tension. Breathe very softly and evenly.

When you feel something at the base of the spine, perhaps heat or a tingling sensation, expand that feelling as much as you can to your back, arms, head, and your whole body. However, if you feel strong heat rising up your spine, do not continue the exercise; instead, gently lower your arms, straighten your head, and remain in the sitting posture for five to ten minutes, expanding the sensations in your body.

After holding the position for three to five minutes, slowly lower your arms to your sides, straighten your head, and stand relaxed for several minutes, expanding the sensations in your body. Do the exercise three times, standing relaxed after each repetition. Then sit in the sitting posture for five to ten minutes, continuing to expand the feelings activated by the exercise.

A variation of this exercise is done with the knees bent. Experiment to see how feeling is affected by different degrees of bending in the knees.

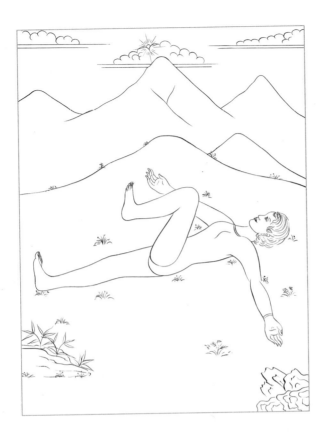

Exercise 92   Channeling Body Energy into the Senses

This exercise is a little strenuous; if you are an older person unused to regular exercise, it is best to skip this one.

Lie on your back with your arms stretched out to your sides at shoulder height, the palms facing up. Separate your legs the width of your pelvis and flex your ankles so that the toes of both feet point toward your head. Sliding your heel along the floor until it lifts naturally, bend your left knee and bring your thigh as close as possible to your torso, keeping the right leg straight. Draw your thigh toward your body, in a strong movement. Breathing through both nose and mouth, hold the tension in legs and feet for fifteen to thirty seconds, keeping your arms and shoulders relaxed. Then very slowly release the tension, straighten your leg and relax your feet, expanding the sensations stimulated by producing and releasing tension in this way. Rest for a moment on your back.

Now flex your ankles, bend your right knee, bring the thigh close to your torso, and repeat the exercise. Do the complete exercise, first on one side, then the other, three times, resting for a few minutes after each repetition. When you finish, rest on your back for five to ten minutes, keeping the arms outstretched at shoulder height, palms up, and continue to amplify and extend the sensations in your body.

A variation of this exercise is done with both thighs pressed to the body at once; this version may produce more intense feelings.

Stage Three

These exercises are more advanced than those in Stages One and Two. Some are physically strenuous; in others a quality of concentration is needed to develop the feeling-tones that are stimulated. Therefore, it is best to wait until you have deepened your experience of Kum Nye over a period of several months before trying these exercises.

When you feel ready, add one or two of these exercises to your practice. Do not push yourself, however, and wait until you have had even more experience before trying the last ten exercises.

If you have not already done so, you might now want to practice some of the exercises at different tempos. Begin with one that you know well and try it in different ways. First do it slowly, and then, without losing touch with the feeling-tones, build up some speed. Then develop the different feeling-tones generated at various tempos.

You will find that all the exercises done tensely can be done in a relaxed way, and those done 'loosely' can also be done tensely. As awareness of subtle inner feelings grows, you will discover how to use both tempo and tension to strengthen and expand the feeling-tones of each exercise.

Let your practice of Kum Nye yoga be an open-ended journey into your inner senses and feelings. As your body and mind become more integrated, your experience of greater balance will itself become your guide.

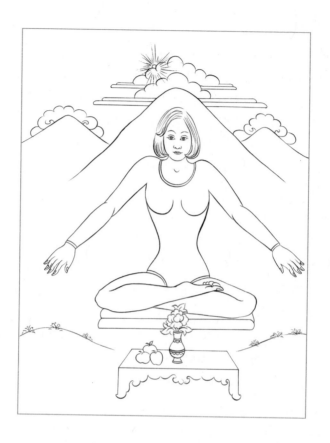

Exercise 93   Refreshing the Senses

Sit cross-legged on a mat or cushion with your hands
on your knees and your back straight. Slowly lift your
arms away from your sides to shoulder height, with the
palms facing behind you. Then lower them until they
are at about a forty-five degree angle from your body.
Lift your shoulders as high as possible, and tuck your
chin in a little. In this position, imagine that a person
who is stronger than you is pushing against your hands

358

and arms, forcing them backward. Maintain tension in hands and arms, relax your belly and lower back, and slowly move your hands and arms back and up. It is not necessary to go very far back or up. With your body still, your chest open, and your spine balanced, hold this position for one minute or ten to fifteen out breaths. Breathe gently and evenly through both nose and mouth.

Release the tension as slowly as you can, sensing the feelings generated by holding in this way. Then bring your hands to your knees and rest a minute, letting the ripples of sensation move through and beyond the body. Do the exercise three times, resting briefly after each repetition. At the end, remain sitting for five to ten minutes. Continue to expand the feelings that have been stimulated during this exercise.

This exercise releases both physical and psychological tension, and stimulates the flow of sensation throughout the whole body.

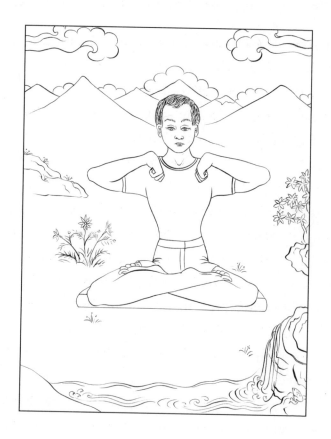

Exercise 94   Nurturing Body Energy

Sit cross-legged on a mat or cushion and run the fingers along your collarbone until you feel it meet the bone of your shoulder. Make light fists with your fingers and press the thumbs gently into the depressions on the lower side of the collarbone. With your mouth open slightly, breathing evenly through nose and mouth, slowly jut out your jaw. As you do so, gradually increase the pressure of your thumbs until the pressure is quite strong.

Hold for one to three minutes, going deeply into your sensations. Notice the quality of your breath, for it will reveal your emotional state. Allow whatever emotions or sensations you feel to come to the surface.

Then very slowly release the tension in your thumbs, neck, and jaw, allowing your sensations to fill the field of experience. Sit quietly for several minutes with your hands on your knees, expanding your feelings throughout your body. Now repeat the exercise. If you find primitive sounds arising within you, perhaps expressions of rage or pain, express them. You may want to make sounds during the entire period of holding.

Again, very slowly release the tension, and sit quietly for several minutes. Observe. What are the qualities of your breathing? What is your state of mind?

Do the exercise three or nine times, resting for a few minutes after each repetition and for five to ten minutes at the end.

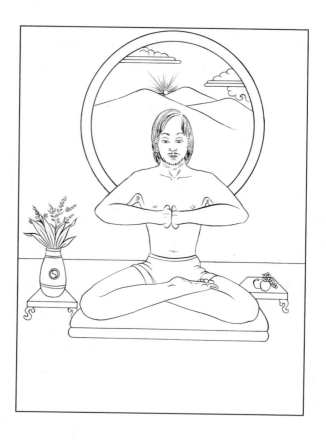

Exercise 95   Stimulating Inner Energy

This exercise is especially effective when done after massaging the back of the neck.

Sit cross-legged on a mat or cushion, press your palms together, and turn your hands so your fingertips touch the center of your chest. As you inhale, push inward and a little upward (do this more with the breath than with the hands). Stretch your neck upward, with your chin tucked in. Now hold your breath, press your chin strongly in, and inwardly make a push to the back of your neck. You may feel sensations of warmth in that area. Continue holding your breath for as long as you can, and expand your sensations, letting them flow down your spine and spread throughout your body.

Now slowly exhale and release the tension, letting the subtle inner feelings radiate throughout your whole body and spread to the environment. Let the boundaries between inner and outer spaces melt. Continue to sit for several minutes, quietly sensing the feelings within and around you. Do the exercise three or nine times, sitting after each repetition and at the end.

Certain positions produce certain energies. In this particular exercise, a positive energy builds up until it nurtures the whole body.

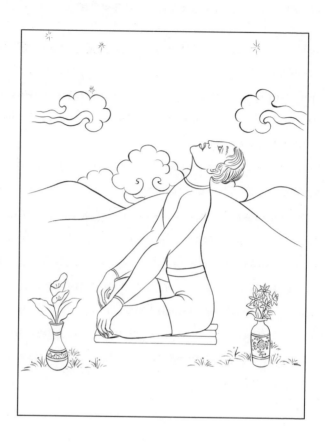

Exercise 96   Wholeness of Joy

Do this exercise very gently if you are pregnant, if you have had any sort of back or neck injury, or if you have had an operation within three or four months.

Sit cross-legged on a mat or cushion or on a low stool with your back straight. Grasp the knees strongly for support and lift your chest toward the ceiling. Be sure to hold your knees firmly with your hands, until there is a feeling of strength in your arms, knees, and hands. As your back arches, open your mouth and carefully let the chin move toward the ceiling. Be sure that the head does not go all the way back, for too extreme a curve in the neck will interrupt the flow of sensation. Breathe softly and evenly through both nose and mouth. Relax your belly; this will make it possible to stretch the spine backward a little more, but be careful not to strain. Hold this position for one to three minutes, sensing the feelings in your chest and spine.

When you feel heat warming the back of your neck, very gradually move forward, straightening your spine. As you release the tension, be aware of sensations of heat and energy that may extend beyond the ordinary limits of your body. You may feel a deep joy. Repeat the exercise three or nine times, resting in the sitting posture for a few minutes after each repetition and for five to ten minutes at the end.

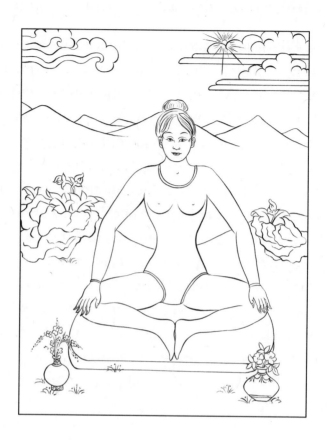

Exercise 97   Touching Time

Sit on a mat or cushion, place the soles of the feet together, and draw them as close to your body as possible. Put your hands on your kneecaps, lift your elbows a little, and press down. Both elbows should be at the same height, and your shoulders level as well. In this position, stretch your upper back up a little, and settle your neck down between your shoulders. Then very slowly bend forward from the waist as low as you can, relaxing the thigh socket as much as possible. Stay down for one to three minutes, breathing gently through both nose and mouth. Then gradually straighten your spine, feeling the sensations in your body. If staying down is too difficult, then slowly straighten your spine without holding. Rest briefly, expanding the sensations quickened by the exercise.

Do the exercise three or nine times, sitting quietly for a few minutes after each repetition and for five to ten minutes at the end, continuing to expand the sensations within and around your body.

This exercise will stretch the thigh and back muscles, releasing energies held in the thigh socket, the sacrum, and the spine.

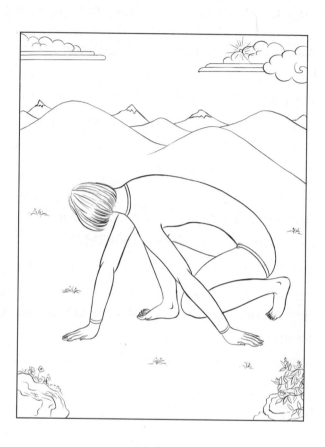

Exercise 98   Inner Immortality of Energy

Kneel on your left knee and place your right foot flat on the floor just in front of the left knee, so the heel and knee touch. Lift your left foot a little and stand on your left toes; then sit all the way back so your left buttock rests on your left ankle. Be alert and sensitive to the left toes during the exercise, so you do not put too much weight on them. If they become painful, straighten the foot so the toes point behind you and do the exercise that way.

Place the hands on the floor to the left of your body, widely separated, with the fingers of the right hand pointing in the same direction as the right foot, and the fingers of the left hand pointing in the opposite direction. Keeping both arms straight, twist head and torso to the right, so your left shoulder moves down and your right shoulder moves up a little. Look up toward the ceiling, with your chin near your right shoulder. Breathe evenly through both nose and mouth and feel the sensations produced by this twist in your spine. Hold for thirty seconds to one minute.

To change your position so you can do the twist to the left, slowly straighten your neck and let your head hang down in a relaxed way; then slide your hands along the floor toward each other until they are about a foot apart, with the fingers pointing left (left in relation to your body). Standing on your left toes, lift your left knee and swing it a little to the left, then lift your right heel so you stand also on your right toes, and swivel both feet until they point in the same direction as your hands. Lower your head and lift your pelvis toward the ceiling until your legs are almost straight. Swivel your toes to the left, kneel on your right knee, place your left heel in front of your right knee, and separate your hands, pointing the fingers of the left hand in the same direction as the left foot and the fingers of the right hand in the opposite direction. In this position, keeping your arms straight and breathing gently through both nose and mouth, do the spinal twist to the left.

Do the complete exercise, twisting first to one side, then to the other, three times. Then sit in the sitting posture for five to ten minutes, expanding the sensations stimulated by this movement.

Exercises 99 through 102 stimulate joyful feelings, activate sexual energies and distribute them throughout the body. They relieve negative patterns, such as resistance, and vitalize inner energies. In all of these exercises, the muscles of the backs of the legs are stretched. In most people, these muscles are quite contracted, so be sensitive and alert when doing an exercise not to stretch too much. The exercises will be effective with even a slight stretch. For older persons who are not used to regular exercise, it may be best not to attempt these exercises. In any case, do them gently, slowly easing into the stretch and developing a quality of lightness.

Explore each exercise fully before trying another. Try not to be in a rush. Each exercise stimulates slightly different feeling-tones, and it is possible to become sensitive to the subtle flavors of each. You do not need to do these exercises in the sequence presented here.

You may feel more, and be less likely to stretch too much, if you massage the backs of your legs before doing an exercise. For the massage, lie on your back, bend your knees one at a time, and place your feet flat on the floor. Bring your right knee close to your chest, straighten the leg toward the ceiling, supporting the back of the thigh with interlaced hands. Move the leg back and forth slowly and lightly a few times. Then gently point first the toe and then the heel to the ceiling three or four times.

Now lock your leg straight with the foot parallel to the ceiling, and grasp the back of the thigh with both hands so your fingers meet in the middle. Massage the back of the thigh firmly in horizontal strokes, working from the center out to the sides. Work up the back of the leg toward the foot, lifting your head if necessary to help you reach the lower leg. Breathe gently through both nose and mouth as you stroke, letting the breath merge with both motion and sensation.

When you finish, slowly bend the right knee and lower the right foot to the floor. Rest for a few minutes, expanding the sensations generated by the massage. Then repeat the massage for the left leg.

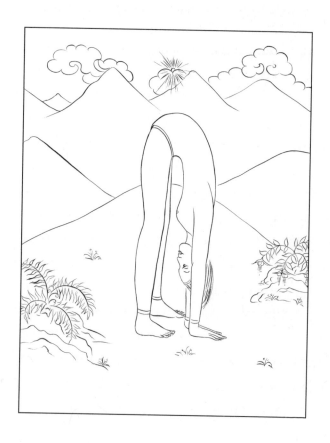

Exercise 99   Touching Positive Feeling

With your feet a few inches apart, squat on the toes and balls of your feet. With your arms outside of your legs, place the palms flat on the floor in front of you, the fingers pointing forward. Look up toward the ceiling, breathing gently through nose and mouth.

Keeping your palms flat on the floor, slowly lower your head, lift the pelvis toward the ceiling as far as you can without straining, and lower your heels to the floor.

Feel the stretch in the backs of your legs, making sure not to stretch too much. Hold for thirty seconds to one minute, relaxing your feet and belly, letting your head hang loosely from your neck, and breathing as evenly as possible through both nose and mouth. If your legs tremble or shake, go into the shaking and release tensions.

Now slowly lower your pelvis, lift your head and heels, squat briefly on the toes and balls of your feet. Then sit in the sitting posture for one to two minutes, expanding the sensations stimulated by the leg stretch. You may feel warmth moving up your legs into your pelvis. Expand these sensations to your spine, your upper body, your arms and head. Feel them more. Let them permeate every cell in your whole body.

Do the exercise three times, sitting after each repetition and for five to ten minutes at the end, expanding and distributing the feelings awakened by the exercise.

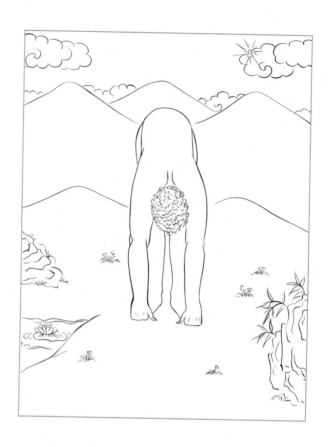

Exercise 100 Wholesome Energy

With your feet a few inches apart, squat on the toes and balls of your feet. Make fists, and with your arms outside your legs, place the first and second knuckles of the fists flat on the floor. Then place the thumbs flat on the floor, pointing toward each other.

Keeping your fists and thumbs on the floor, lower your head, lift the pelvis toward the ceiling as high as you can without straining, and lower your heels to the floor.

Remember to ease into the stretch in a light and gentle way. (If you find it too difficult to straighten your legs, do not be concerned. When you stay with your sensations and continue to relax subtle tensions, the exercise will be effective.) When your pelvis is as high as it can comfortably be. look up and hold this position for thirty seconds to one minute, breathing gently through both nose and mouth. Concentrate lightly on your feelings.

After thirty seconds to one minute, slowly lower your head, lower your pelvis, lift your heels, squat briefly on the toes and balls of your feet, and then sit quietly for one to two minutes, expanding the feelings quickened by the leg stretch.

Do the exercise three times, sitting still after each repetition and for five to ten minutes at the end, expanding the sensations within and around your body.

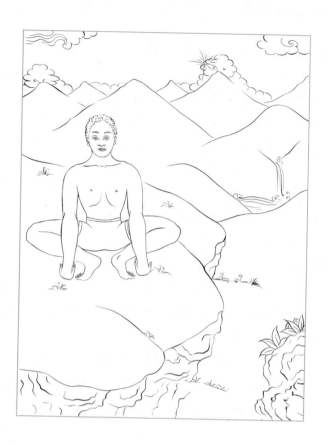

Exercise 101   Touching Present Energy

With your feet apart about the width of your pelvis, squat on the toes and balls of your feet and widely separate your knees.

Turn your arms so the inner arm faces forward and the fingers point behind you. With your arms inside your legs, place the hands flat on the floor a little further apart than your feet. Look straight ahead, with your chest as high as possible.

Keeping your hands flat on the floor, slowly lower your head, lift your pelvis as high as you can without straining, and lower your heels to the floor. Relax your neck and let your head hang. Feel the stretch in the backs of your legs and in your arms, but be sure not to stretch too much. Stay in this position for thirty seconds to one minute, breathing evenly through both nose and mouth and relaxing your feet and belly. If your legs shake, go into the shaking and release as much tension as you can.

Slowly lower your pelvis, lifting your heels, and lifting your head. Then squat briefly on the toes and balls of your feet holding your chest high. Finally remain in the sitting posture for one to two minutes, expanding the sensations quickened by the stretch.

Do the exercise three times, sitting for a few minutes after each repetition and for five to ten minutes at the end, continuing to amplify the feelings that are within and around your body.

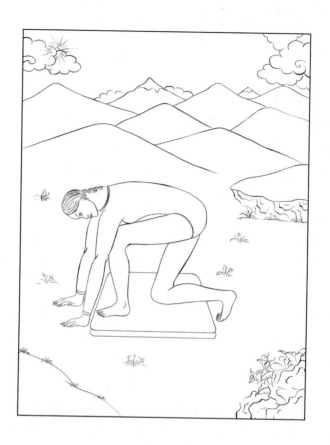

Exercise 102   Texture of Joy

Get down on your hands and knees, with a pillow under just the knees. Point your fingers forward. Lift your feet a little and stand on your toes, so your weight is balanced on your toes, knees, and hands. Keeping your palms flat on the floor and your arms straight, slowly lower your head, shift your weight forward a little, and lift your knees until your legs are straight. Then lower your heels to the ground. Hold this stretch for thirty seconds to one minute, breathing gently through both nose and mouth, and feeling the sensations in the backs of your legs. Let your head hang loosely from your neck. If you cannot bring your heels all the way to the ground, lower them as far as you can without straining the muscles of the backs of your legs, and hold the stretch in this position. Bringing your hands closer to your body will also decrease the stretch. In time you may find that you can bring your heels all the way to the floor.

After thirty seconds to a minute, very slowly bend your knees and lower them to the pillow, sensing the feelings stimulated in your body as you release the stretch. Rest briefly on your hands and knees with your feet relaxed, soles up, continuing to expand the sensations quickened by the movement. Do the exercise three times, resting briefly after each repetition. At the end, sit in the sitting posture for five to ten minutes, continuing to expand the sensations produced by the exercise.

The following version of this exercise is a little more strenuous. To take the position illustrated in the drawing, kneel on a mat and locate a spot about one foot in front of your left knee. Lift your left leg and place your left foot on that spot. Lift your right foot a little and stand on the toes. Then place your palms flat on the floor in front of you, a shoulder width apart, with your fingers pointing forward.

Now keeping your palms flat on the floor, slowly lower your head, lift your right knee, and lower your right heel to the floor, straightening both legs as much possible. Hold the stretch for thirty seconds to one minute. Be sure to keep your palms flat on the floor. Then slowly bend your right knee and lower it to the mat, feeling the sensations released in the body. Rest briefly on hands and knees, with your feet relaxed, soles up.

Now reverse the position of your legs and repeat the exercise. Do the complete movement, first on one side, then on the other, three times, resting briefly after each stretch. At the end, sit in the sitting posture for five to ten minutes, allowing the feelings stimulated by this exercise to be distributed throughout your body, and also beyond it to the surrounding environment.

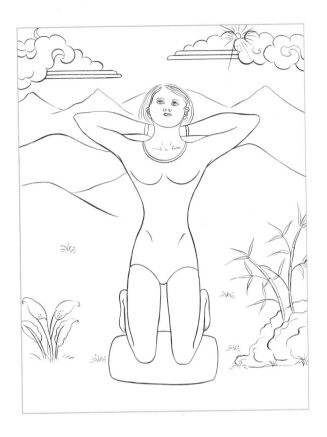

Exercise 103 Vitality

Kneel on a mat or soft pillow with your thighs vertical.
Lift your feet a little and stand on your toes, being careful
not to put too much pressure on them. (For some people
the posture will be difficult, with the toes in this position.
If this is the case, straighten your feet so the toes point
backward, and do the exercise that way.) Interlace your
fingers and place them at the back of your neck, with the
elbows wide apart.

In this position, breathing gently through both nose and mouth, very slowly arch backward without straining, and hold for fifteen to thirty seconds. Feel sensations in the small of your back, and relax your throat, chest, and belly as much as possible.

Then very slowly—it is important to move very slowly throughout this exercise—straighten your spine and sit back on your heels. Then lifting first one knee and then the other, squat on the toes and balls of your feet with your heels together. Spread your knees wide apart and slowly bend forward as far as possible, keeping the elbows wide apart. Let your head hang loosely from your neck.

Hold for fifteen to thirty seconds, breathing easily through both nose and mouth, feeling the sensations in your spine. Then slowly straighten back up, bringing your knees closer together, and moving from squatting to kneeling (kneel first on one knee and then on the other). Sowly raise your pelvis until your thighs are more or less vertical. Then slowly arch backward, beginning the movement once again.

Except for the two points of holding, this exercise is done as a continuous movement. Do the exercise *very slowly* three times, breathing easily through both nose and mouth, and concentrating lightly on the sensations in your spine. To complete the exercise, sit in the sitting posture for five to ten minutes, expanding the sensations within and around your body.

A variation of this exercise is done with the hands clasped at the back of the head. Notice the different sensations produced by the different stretch.

This exercise will revitalize the whole body, increase stability, and improve coordination.

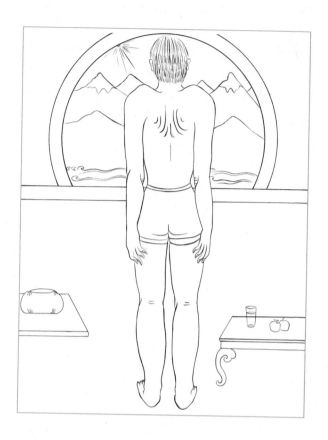

Exercise 104   Sacred Energy

Stand well balanced with your feet a comfortable distance
apart, the back straight and the arms relaxed at your sides.
Move your shoulders back as far as you can, squeezing
your shoulder blades together. When you think you have
moved your shoulders back as far as possible, move them
back more. Now move them backward a little more, until
you almost feel thick wrinkles in the skin of your back,
between the shoulder blades.

Keeping your shoulders back, lift them a little, and grasp your thighs with your hands. Your back, arms, and shoulders should be very tense. Relax your chin and settle your neck down, in between your shoulders. Hold this position for one to three minutes, breathing gently through both nose and mouth, with the front of your body as relaxed as possible. Relax your thighs.

Now without hurrying release the tension—take about one minute for this—and stand with your arms relaxed at your sides for one to two minutes, letting subtle qualities of feeling spread throughout your body. Do the exercise three times, standing in a relaxed way after each repetition. To complete the exercise, sit in the sitting posture for five to ten minutes, allowing the feelings quickened by the movement to expand.

This exercise stimulates heat that moves to the inner core of the body and balances the energies of the front and back of the body.

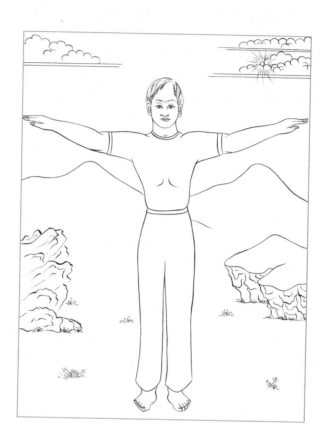

Exercise 105　Heart Gold Thread

Stand well balanced with your feet about six inches apart, your back straight, and your arms relaxed at your sides. Slowly lift the arms away from your sides to just above shoulder height, with the palms down. Bend the elbows very slightly. Close your eyes and bring your awareness and concentration to your heart center. Sense the heart pumping blood throughout your body; then expand and deepen your awareness, sending the energy of the heart center outward through your arms. Breathe very lightly and evenly, through both nose and mouth. Standing very still, hold this position for ten minutes. After two or three minutes, slightly loosen the muscles on the top of your shoulder joint; this may make the position easier to hold.

After ten minutes, lower your arms very slowly and gently, taking about one minute to lower them all the way down to your sides. Stand silently with your arms at your sides for a few minutes, expanding the sensations generated by this posture. Then lie down on your back for ten minutes, continuing to amplify these sensations until they spread even beyond your body.

This exercise balances the heart center, increases mental and physical energy, improves circulation (and the complexion), and builds strength and concentration. The exercise can also be an instrument for identifying and transforming psychological and physical blockages. As you do it, notice weak or tense areas of your body; notice also the times at which you lose strength and focus, and want to give up. If you feel fear or pain, bring this feeling into your heart center and touch it with concentration and awareness.

A memory of an emotion may come into your mind, perhaps sorrow, hurt, or pain. Expand the feeling, letting senses and mind become one. Stay with the feeling until you penetrate it, and release it into pure experience. A flash of energy—the energy of that memory—then enters the present, and the pattern of the emotion melts and no longer exists. Then you will be beyond pain, surrounded by an expressive quality which means you are no longer holding—a quality of 'here I am' which can be observed and felt in every cell of your body.

You feel a sense of union, a willingness to let feelings arise and expand, and you are able to embrace experience directly, without hesitation. With more experience, it is possible to face pain, fear, and tension directly, letting them go as they occur in daily life.

As you become familiar with this exercise, try holding the position for longer periods of time, up to twenty-five minutes. Rest afterwards for as long as you held the position, standing and then lying down, or, first if you wish, simply lying down.

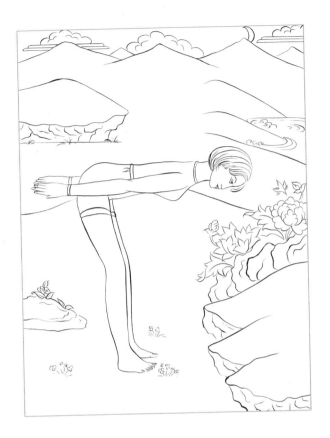

Exercise 106 Trinity of Practice: Breath, Energy, and Awareness

Stand well balanced with your feet a few inches apart, your back straight, and arms relaxed at your sides. Extend your arms in front of you, palms together, with the fingers pointing straight ahead.

In one flowing, continuous movement, stretch your arms forward and push your pelvis backward, lowering the head between your arms, until your torso, head, and arms are parallel to the ground. Keep your back straight throughout this movement.

In this position, stretch forward with the arms and at the same time, stretch the pelvis backward. The knees are straight. Do not hold your breath; breathe as evenly as you can through both nose and mouth. Interlace the fingers and stretch more, in both directions; your body will lower a little. Stretch even more, until you feel you have touched a place of energy. You may begin to shake. Hold this position for fifteen to thirty seconds.

Now, without releasing the tension, very slowly move your hands apart, and keeping your arms at the same level, move them in an arc, palms down, until they are straight in back of you and close to your body. In this position, stretch your neck forward and push your pelvis backward until you feel the energy. Hold the posture as long as you can, breathing evenly through both nose and mouth.

Then slowly release the tension and stand up, carrying your weight in your legs. Stand silently for three to five minutes and then repeat the exercise twice, resting after each repetition. Then sit in the sitting posture for fifteen minutes, broadening the sensations until they spread out to the universe and you are aware of nothing else. You may feel openings along the spine and in your chest, hands, neck, and head.

This exercise stimulates and revitalizes inner energies and builds strength and concentration.

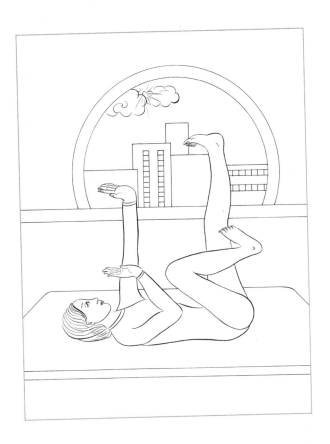

Exercise 107   Expanding Inner Energy

Lie down on your back with your legs a comfortable distance apart and your arms at your sides. Bend your knees, one at a time, and bring them close to your chest. Flex your ankles so the toes point toward your head. (They will stay this way throughout the exercise.) Slide your arms along the floor until they are stretched out at shoulder height, with the palms up. In this position, draw your thighs strongly toward your torso. When you do this, you will feel the muscle in the top of the thigh which controls this movement. Relax your shoulders, neck, and arms, and breathe gently through both nose and mouth.

Now while still keeping your left thigh as close to your body as you can, slowly extend your right leg (with the ankle flexed) toward the ceiling. Feel the contraction in the left thigh and the extension in the right. Then bend the right knee and bring the right thigh as close to your body as you can, and at the same time extend the left leg toward the ceiling. Keep your upper body and your belly as relaxed as possible throughout the movement. Let breath and awareness expand your sensations and become one with the movement.

Do the complete movement (including both sides of the body) three continuous times. Then slowly lower the left leg, release the tension, and one at a time, bring your feet back to the floor and straighten your legs. Rest on your back for five to ten minutes, expanding the sensations that have been stimulated by this movement.

When you become familiar with the above exercise, try this variation: lie on your back with your legs a comfortable distance apart and your arms close to your body, bent at the elbows so your palms face the ceiling. Bend your knees one at a time and bring them close to your chest. Flex your ankles so the toes point toward your head. Imagine that a strong force is pushing against your hands, creating tension in your arms as well as in your legs.

Maintaining the tension in your left arm and leg, slowly extend both your right arm (with the palm parallel to the ceiling) and your right leg (with the ankel flexed) toward the ceiling. Then slowly bend and lower the right arm and leg, bringing them close to your body, and at the same time extend the left arm and leg.

Do the complete movement (including both sides of the body) three continuous times. Then slowly begin to lower the left arm and leg and slowly release the tension in both arms and legs. Bring your feet back to the floor one at a time, straighten your legs, and bring your arms to your sides.

Rest on your back for five to ten minutes, breathing gently and evenly through nose and mouth, expanding the sensations awakened by this movement.

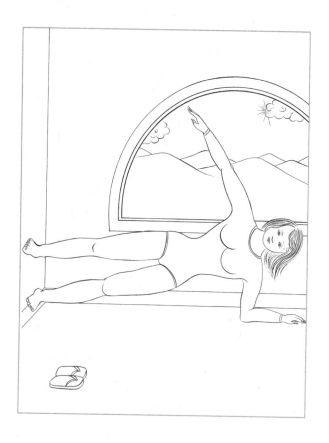

Exercise 108 Touching the Present Body

Find a smooth wall with plenty of space in front of it. Lie down on your left side with your left arm overhead on the floor, the palm down. Rest your head on your arm, and with the legs straight, place both feet flat against the wall, about six inches apart, with the left foot next to the floor. Support yourself with your right palm on the floor near your chest, raise the head and upper torso, and bend the left arm at the elbow, bringing your elbow closer to your body until the bend in the elbow makes a right angle, and your forearm is resting on the floor, with the palm down. Then rest your right arm along the right side of your body.

In this position, breathing gently through both nose and mouth, push your left foot against the wall, and lift your left leg and hip off the floor. The right leg stays relatively relaxed. Hold a few seconds, then slowly bring your hip and leg back to the floor and rest briefly, expanding the feelings stimulated in your body. Notice the quality of your breathing. Then roll slowly onto your right side, and repeat the movement, this time pushing the right foot against the wall.

Do the complete exercise, first on one side and then on the other, three times, resting briefly after each side. At the end, lie on your back and rest in this position for five to ten minutes, continuing to expand the sensations awakened by this movement.

A variation of this exercise is to lift the upper arm until it points toward the ceiling as you lift the hip and leg.

This exercise relieves qualities of inner holding and inner chill and creates lightness in the body.

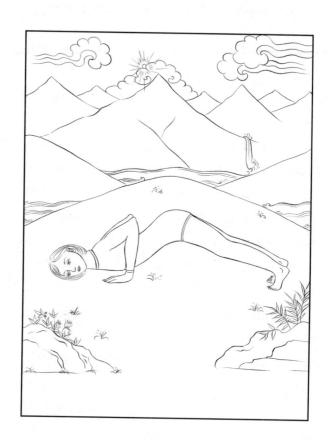

Exercise 109   Wholeness of Energy

Lie on your stomach with your legs a comfortable distance
apart and your face turned to one side, with the cheek
resting on the floor.

Stand on your toes and place your palms flat on the
floor near your chest, with the elbows up. Keeping your
chest on the floor, lift your pelvis as high as you can without straining; walking your toes toward your pelvis will
help to lift it higher. Be sure not to put too much pressure

on your neck. Hold the pelvis up for fifteen to thirty seconds, breathing evenly and gently through both nose and mouth.

Then slowly lower your pelvis to the ground, relax your feet, turn your head to the other side, and place your arms at your sides. Rest briefly, expanding the sensations stimulated by this movement. Do the exercise three times, resting on your stomach after each repetition. At the end, roll over onto your back, bend your knees, bring them close to your chest, and clasp your arms around your knees. Remain in this position for five to ten minutes, continuing to amplify and extend the sensations in your body.

A slightly more difficult version of this exercise is done with the top of the forehead on the floor.

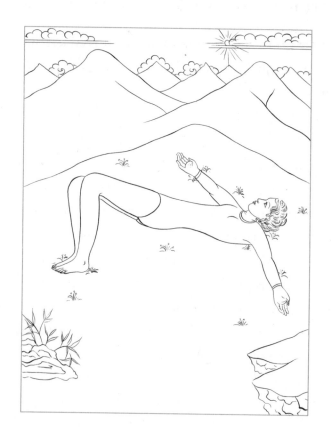

Exercise 110 Energizing Body and Mind

Lie down on your back with your arms extended to your sides at shoulder level, the palms up. Bend your knees slightly, bring your feet together with the foot soles on the floor, and open your knees as wide as possible. Be sure that most of the sole of the foot stays on the floor, although the inside of the foot will lift slightly. Now lift the pelvis as high as you can, so your weight rests on your shoulders and feet. Breathing softly through both nose and mouth, hold this position one to three minutes. Your legs and pelvis may quake a little. Be mindful of any changes in your breathing.

After one to three minutes, slowly lower your pelvis to the floor, straighten your legs one at a time, and bring your arms to your sides. Rest for a few minutes, expanding the feelings stimulated by this exercise. You may feel heat between the shoulder blades and sensations of opening or clarity in the lower energy centers. Do the exercise three times, resting after each repetition. At the end, draw your knees toward your chest, put your hands on your knees, and rest in this position for five to ten minutes.

• A variation of this exercise is to lift the chest instead of the pelvis. Lie on your back with your arms relaxed at your sides, your knees slightly bent, and your feet together.

Open your knees wide, keeping your feet as flat on the floor as possible. While lifting your chest with the help of your elbows, bend your head back so you can rest the top of your head on the floor. Then stretch your arms out to your sides at shoulder level, with the palms up.

Hold this position for one to three minutes, breathing easily through both nose and mouth. Then very slowly bring your arms to your sides and support your weight on your forearms, straighten your neck, lower your back to the floor, and straighten your legs one at a time. Rest for several minutes, expanding the sensations stimulated by this exercise. You may feel sensations of opening in the chest. Do the exercise three times, resting after each repetition. Remain still for five to ten minutes at the end.

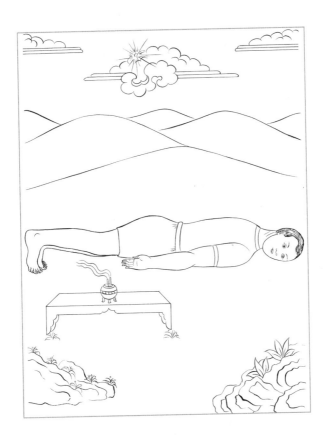

Exercise 111 Circulating Energy

The position for this exercise is somewhat delicate, and requires a subtle kind of balance; you will find it easier to do some days than on others. Lie down on the floor on your stomach, with your legs slightly apart, your arms at your sides, and your head turned to one side. Lift your feet a little and stand on your toes. In this position, gently raise your knees, thighs, and lower abdomen (up to about four inches below the navel) an inch or more above the floor.

Your upper torso remains in contact with the floor. There will be some tension in your hips and in the area of the sacrum, but your chest, shoulders, and throat should be relaxed, and your breathing easy and effortless through both nose and mouth. As much as possible, relax also the backs of your legs.

Tighten your belly slightly and hold your breath back a little, directly in front of the sacrum; this will help to generate energy. Concentrate lightly on the base of your spine. As soon as you feel a sensation there—perhaps warmth or a delicious kind of healing energy—slightly increase the tension in your sacral area. Keep your knees straight. Do not tighten too much—if you do, breathing in the chest will become difficult, you will have to breathe quickly and heavily, and the energy will become clouded and diminish. You need to find a place of balance, not strained and not too loose; then certain feelings are generated within the body. Your chest and throat should be relaxed, the area beneath the navel (both front and back) a little tense, and your breath light.

Once you feel the energy flowing in this circular path and are able to maintain it, hold the position for three to five minutes. Then gently sink to the floor and rest for three to five minutes, continuing to breathe in the same rhythm as before. Turn the head to the other side if you wish. Then again elevate your legs and lower stomach and continue the turning of the energy wheel for five to fifteen minutes.

If you are not able to contact this energy, separate your knees slightly—this automatically creates a little more tension in your first and second energy centers, generating more energy which then moves to the back of the sacrum where you can feel it. At the moment the energy goes to the base of the spine, be very careful not to tighten your chest. Your chest should be loose and almost still. If you do not experience this energy physically, then imagine it; you can discover a very joyful and refreshing feeling.

If you have difficulty lifting your lower body from the floor, do not strain but just breathe very subtly, holding your breath a tiny bit in your stomach and at the back of your spine near the sacrum. Imagine the lower body lifting as if drawn up by a magnet. If you breathe too heavily, you will not be able to feel the energy flow in your spine. Loosen your stomach—very heavy tension there can also make this position difficult.

Should you have difficulty holding your legs and the lower energy centers off the floor for the entire duration of five to fifteen minutes, then lift them up for a shorter time, even a few seconds. Let your lower back be as loose as it can be in this position. If you find it difficult to lift your knees, then stretch your legs as if to lengthen them, and the knees will come off the floor. If, however, you still cannot hold the posture, let your knees touch the floor, making sure that the lower energy centers do not press to the ground heavily.

If you are unable to hold this position at all, just lie on your stomach and be very relaxed. Feel the energy rising from behind the base of the spinal cord, moving forward to the lower part of the stomach and up into your chest. Feel the flow of energy relaxing your chest and throat. Follow the energy up inside your head and back under the skull to the spinal cord. Warm energy rises there, and passes slowly down the whole length of your spine.

Resting afterwards is an integral part of the exercise. Sink slowly to the ground and rest on your stomach for at least as long as you have held the position, experiencing the movement of feeling and energy within you. After resting, roll onto your side, bend your knees, draw them up toward your chest, and slowly come up to a sitting position, supporting yourself with one hand on the floor. This exercise may affect your sense of time, and it is important to move very slowly, and with awareness, as you sit and stand. Before standing, move your head slowly up and down and from side to side to relieve any tenseness there.

This exercise releases energy blockages (including sexual blockages) in the lower energy centers and distributes this energy throughout the body.

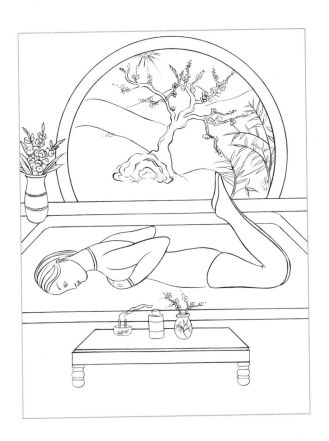

Exercise 112 Stimulating Balanced Energy

Lie on your stomach with your face turned to the left and
your cheek resting on the floor. Separate your legs a comfortable distance apart, bend your knees, point your toes to
the ceiling, and bring your heels close to your buttocks.

Place the top of your forehead on the floor and put
your palms on either side of your chest, so your fingers
meet in the center of the chest. Keeping your forehead
on the floor, use your hands and arms to slowly lift your

chest as high as possible off the floor without straining. Hold this position for about thirty seconds to one minute, breathing evenly and gently through both nose and mouth.

Now sink back to the floor, while slowly releasing the tension. Turn your head to the right side, straighten your legs, bring your arms to your sides, and rest briefly in this position, amplifying the sensations that were stimulated by this movement. You may feel warmth in your chest and tingling sensations in your lower back.

Do the movement three times, resting on your stomach after each repetition. At the end, roll onto your back, bend your knees and bring them to your chest, clasp your arms around your knees, and rest for five to ten minutes, continuing to expand the feelings. If you wish, straighten your legs and rest your arms at your sides.

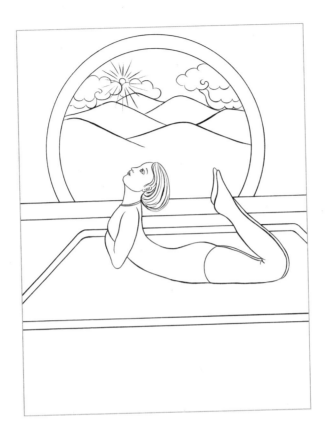

Exercise 113   Tasting Bliss

Lie on your stomach with your head turned to one side,
your legs a comfortable distance apart, and your arms at
your sides. Bend both your knees, and point your toes
toward the ceiling.

Place the top of your forehead on the floor and put
your left palm on the left side of your chest and your right
palm on the right side of your chest, so the fingers meet in
the center of the chest.

Now move your feet in the direction of your head, and your head in the direction of your feet, so the spine arches backward. Do not strain—move only so far as you can without forcing. Hold a few seconds, then gently return your body to the floor. Turn your head to the other side, straighten your legs, and relax your feet; bring your arms to your sides, and rest for a few minutes.

Repeat the movement three times, using the resting period after each repetition to allow the feelings stimulated by the exercise to expand throughout your body. At the end, roll onto your back, bend the knees and bring them to your chest, clasp your arms around your knees, and rest for five to ten minutes, continuing to expand the sensations within and around the body. If you wish, straighten your legs, and rest both your arms at your sides after a while.

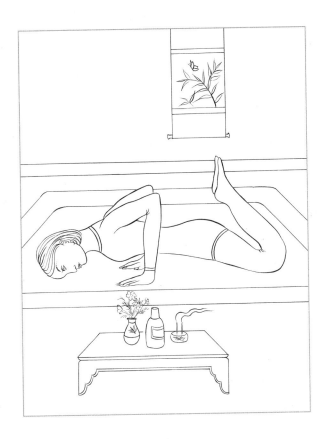

Exercise 114　Utilizing Expansive Energy

Do this exercise on a carpeted floor and put a small pillow under your head. Lie on your stomach and rest the top of your forehead on the pillow.

Place the palms of your hands on the floor near the sides of your chest, with the elbows up and the fingers pointing forward. Separate your legs the width of your pelvis, bend your knees, and point your toes to the ceiling. In this position, push your hands against the floor and lift your torso off the ground as high as you can, so your weight rests on your knees, forehead, and hands. Be sure your forehead stays on the floor. Hold for a few seconds, breathing through both nose and mouth as evenly and gently as you can. If you begin to shake, bring breath and shaking together and release tensions. Then lower your body to the floor, turn your head to one side, straighten the legs, relax the feet, bring your arms to your sides, and rest for a few minutes, expanding the sensations generated by this movement.

Do the exercise three times, resting on your stomach for a few minutes after each repetition, and for five to ten minutes at the end. This exercise may take you to a certain place of intense energy. Feel especially the sensations in your abdomen, perhaps feelings of warmth and a sense of expansion, and distribute them throughout your body.

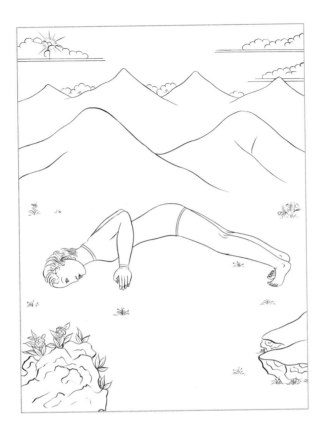

Exercise 115 Wholeness of Body and Mind

Do this exercise barefoot on a carpeted floor, with the help
of a small pillow for your head. Lie on your stomach, the
arms extended to your sides at shoulder level, with the
palms down. Separate your legs a comfortable distance,
and rest the top of your forehead on the pillow. Lift your
feet a little and stand on your toes. Bend your elbows and
slide your hands along the floor toward you until the forearms are vertical. Your fingers will point out sideways.

Now brace your toes against the floor, press your palms and forehead against the floor, and hoist your torso and legs off the floor. Then quickly walk your feet toward your head and roll your head a little, so the top of your head rests on the pillow. Hold for thirty seconds to two minutes, breathing evenly through nose and mouth. Then lower your body to the floor, walking your feet back until you can rest first one leg and then the other on the floor. Turn your head to one side, bring your arms to your sides, and rest for a few minutes, expanding the sensations generated by this movement.

Do the exercise three times, resting briefly after each repetition. At the end, rest a few minutes on your stomach and then roll onto your back and rest for five to ten minutes longer, continuing to extend the feelings within and around your body.

Retreat

Everything you do can be a beautiful ceremony,
a dance of appreciation.

Once or even several times a year, a retreat in a natural setting, however brief, can greatly expand your practice of Kum Nye. Spending four days every season or one week a year in the mountains, or perhaps near the ocean or a river, are beneficial to deepen the Kum Nye relaxation.

During the retreat, be outside as much as you can. In the morning, practice breathing for about an hour. Sit in the sitting posture, gently open your mouth and nostrils, and breathe very, very slowly, holding your belly in a little. Open all your senses as an invitation to the living energies around you to enter your body. Let your whole body, even your toes and hair, sensitively feel the energies of the cosmos—the light, air, earth, plants, water, and sky. Be as sensitive as a fish in water.

Feel the energies flow into you. Visualize the positive healing qualities of all living energies collected in your body. Mix your feelings with these wholesome energies, then let the feelings and energies stream outward from you to the cosmos in an ongoing exercise, a continuing interaction, a circular dance of energy.

Continue this process of healing enjoyment while sunbathing twice a day for about twenty-five minutes (not more than forty minutes at a time). After sunbathing or before sleeping, do an hour of massage, rubbing the oil into your body when you finish. Massaging outside with sesame oil can be an especially delicious experience. During the day, whenever you wish, practice one or two movement exercises you want to develop, and remember OM AH HUM from time to time.

During the time of the retreat, and throughout the year as well, sleep for seven or eight hours a night and eat simple, balanced meals. Do not place too great an emphasis on food, but whatever your diet (and this will depend to some degree on your childhood diet), lighten it a little, and let it be about sixty-five percent or more vegetarian. Vegetables, nuts, and fruits are healthful, as are soybeans; it is best not to eat white flour or sugar. (If you want to pursue the subject of diet, the many books available on nutrition can give you more information.) Chew slowly and thoroughly, enjoying fully the tastes and textures of your food, and leave your stomach half-empty when you finish a meal.

During all of your activities, try to be always relaxed, mindful, and concentrated, bringing the body, the mind, and the senses together. In this way, everything you do can become a beautiful ceremony, and all of your life can be transformed.

Index

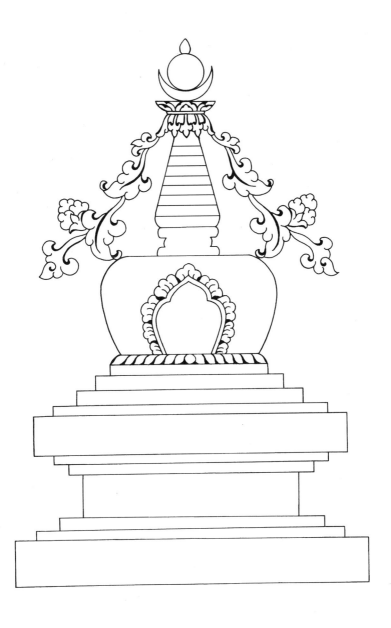

Kum Nye Yoga by email

Kum Nye Yoga classes are also available on Audio CDs (ask for a separate CD catalog) as well as by email, directly from Dharma Publishing Programs. The e-program offers a step-by-step guidance that will help you deepen your practice of Kum Nye Yoga and your understanding of how to live in accord with its basic principles. E-Kum Nye Yoga is offered in multiple languages, including Dutch, English, German, Portuguese and Spanish.

E-Kum Nye Yoga consists of five levels, structured in ten weekly segments. After finishing Level I in ten weeks, you may proceed to Level II. All together, the five levels of e-Kum Nye Yoga provide a year long intensive Kum Nye training.

The Five Levels of e-Kum Nye Yoga:
1 Outer Kum Nye Relaxation: Opening to feeling and to the power of breath.
2 Inner Balance: Integrating body and mind to engender wellness.
3 Transformations: Stimulating and transforming the energies of the four energy centres.
4 The cream of Kum Nye Yoga: Advanced practices to liberate the senses and mind, healing our grasping shadow side.
5 Kum Nye Yoga is life: The joy of being and our offering to the world.

Please join our worldwide *e-Kum Nye Yoga* practice group.

For information please contact us at:
www.kumnyeyoga.com
www.dharmapublishing.com
dp@dharmapublishing.com or visit us at

Authorized Kum Nye Yoga Centers

United States

Nyingma Institute
1815 Highland Place
Berkeley CA 94709
www.nyingmainstitute.com

Center for Kum Nye
North Carolina
4907 Garrett Road
Durham, NC 27707
www.skillfulmeansnc.org

Ratna Ling
Dharma Publishing Programs
35788 Hauser Bridge Road
Cazadero, CA 95421
www.dharmapublishing.com
www.kumnyeyoga.com

Montana Kum Nye Group
PO Box 1865
Bigfork, MT 59911

Germany
Nyingma Zentrum
Deutschland e.V.
Siebachstr. 66
50733 Köln
www.nyingmazentrum.de

The Netherlands
Nyingma Centrum Nederland
Reguliersgracht 25
1017 LJ Amsterdam
www.nyingma.nl

Brazil
Instituto Nyingma do Brasil
Rua Cayowaa, 2 085
01258-011 – Sao Paulo, SP
www.nyingma.com.br

Instituto Nyingma do Rio de
Janeiro
Rua Casuarina - 297
Casa 2 Humaita
22261-160 – Rio de Janeiro, RJ
www.nyingmario.org.br

Argentina
Kum Nye Argentina
Godoy Cruz 1570
Capital Federal,
Buenos Aires – Argentina
kumnye-ar@hotmail.com.ar

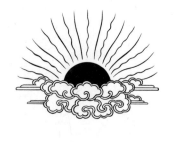